NOTES ON THE NOSODES

TUBERCULINUM
AND
BACILLINUM

By Sheilagh Creasy BAFA,
British Register of
Complementary Practitioners
(Classical Homœopathy)

Notes on the Nosodes
Tuberculinum and Bacillinum

ISBN 0-9525719-0-0

SCHB (Publishing),
29 Lillian Road,
Barnes, London,
SW13 9JG.
ENGLAND.

Edited by: Ralph Varcoe and Noor Khan
Printed by: utl printing
Cover illustration by: Marina Marchione.
Graphics consultant: Nikki Barwood of JB Graphics.

Contents

- 1 -
Introduction to the Nosodes

This booklet is a composition of all the data that I have been able to collect on the subject of Tuberculinum [1]. As a remedy we have very limited writings to turn to and even fewer authors have discussed its role as a nosode in 'unblocking' those cases that won't progress. Facing this gap in my own knowledge led me to seize on any information that I came across on my travels. Many of these notes have therefore come from homœopaths of this century and a proportion from notes of lectures that I actually attended. I have, as far as possible, kept to the original words of the speaker/author but you must, in every case, judge for yourselves the advice which they give. For my own part, I can say that most of what is reported here I have seen in clinical practice. All of the nosodes have their own characteristics and it is important that we study them from all reputable sources.

"The only way, therefore, to use a nosode is to *prove* it on the healthy, like any other drug, and note its symptoms in the regular way." [2] The organisms from tubercular, gonorrheal and syphilitic material give us our remedies of Tuberculinum, Medorrhinum and Syphilinum respectively and potentisation develops their latent dynamic forces; they must therefore be prescribed as conscientiously as any other remedy, all information being found under the provings.

In Hahnemann's organon §203-206, he refers to the venereal diseases and in §206, the complications with psora, which is the most frequent and fundamental cause of chronic disease.

Hahnemann's meaning of the words *"chronic disease"* was that of not only long lasting disease but also a miasm, a disease having a chronic evolution. Miasm is a word which has no translation from the German, the nearest being stigma or taint. I shall use, as a means

1 Where Tuberculinum or Tub is mentioned throughout it refers to Tub Koch or Tub Bov.
2 Allen - Materia Medica of the Nosodes p472, cf. pp295-296.

of describing the underlying constitution, the terms diathesis or dyscrasia, inherent in the individual.

My understanding of the nature of miasms is best illustrated by the following diagram where the line represents time from its beginning to the present day:

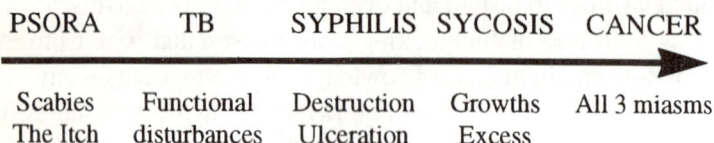

PSORA	TB	SYPHILIS	SYCOSIS	CANCER
Scabies	Functional	Destruction	Growths	All 3 miasms
The Itch	disturbances	Ulceration	Excess	

The Tubercular Dyscrasia

There is a difference of opinion among the various commentators as to whether TB or syphilis was the first to follow psora. The tubercular diathesis is represented, in its early stages, by functional disturbances such as constant colds, headaches and neuralgias which we find in Agaricus, Kali carb, Stannum and China as examples of tubercular remedies. Where these incipient conditions develop then the destructive aspect of the tubercular dyscrasia demonstrates the syphilitic overlay, eg. Drosera with its caries of the bone and Calatropis with its ulceration.

At any time the tubercular tendency (dyscrasia) can be activated by illness, grief, shock or environmental factors, for instance.

Each miasm has its own general character but we frequently find combinations in patients - it is for us to recognise these inherited tendencies, either simple or complex. The recognition and appropriate treatment of such traits in patients before they become parents would remove constitutional encumbrances on future offspring and improve the inborn qualities of a future generation (the science of eugenics).

After Hahnemann it was left to the succeeding homœopathic practitioners to prove the various preparations of Tuberculinum and these notes, compiled from the works of provers and those who added to the original provings by clinical references, form the discussion on the tubercular dyscrasia in this book. All the preparations of Tuberculinum are similar - particular affinities which govern choice in different circumstances are self evident in the notes. When Tuberculinum is requested from the pharmacy it will be supplied as Tuberculinum Koch or Tuberculinum bovinum. Most practitioners find that there is no difference in their actions. If I am disappointed in the action of one then I will make a note so that when Tuberculinum is again indicated in the case I will use the other to see if any greater benefit can be achieved.

The Various Tubercular Preparations

Bacillinum	Proved by Burnett from an extract of human tuberculous sputum.
Tuberculinum Koch	Koch's extracted human tubercle bacilli.
Tuberculinum bovinum	Prepared by Kent from the infected lymph glands of cattle and potentised by Boericke and Taffel.
Tuberculinum denys	Used mostly by Cartier of France and prepared from laboratory cultures.
Marmorek antituberculous	Nebel and Vannier of serum France used this serum in the 6th and 30th potencies.
Tuberculinum aviare	Tuberculin from birds or chicken liver (sources disagree) - used frequently by the French.
Tuberculinum residium	The actual residue left from the preparation of Tuberculinum koch. The French use it frequently.
Bacillinum testium	Prepared from human tuberculous testicles. Proved by Burnett.

- 2 -
Case Evaluation

In the selection of the remedy, one must first and foremost make sure that it is the remedy which is most similar to the evaluated symptom complex of the individual. The patient's story and complaints provide the basis for this, for we are reminded that symptoms are the language of disease. Included would be the history of the person such as late development, enlarged glands, series of bronchial attacks, skin troubles and the general histories of both sides of the family. Kent states that "the disease must be traced in a series from beginning to end and back again, for disease results are according to circumstance and inheritance". In the unravelling of the case a wise injunction is "do not dig too deep too soon" - keep to the uppermost, ie. the most recent development of the patient's disease.

Secondly, in some chronic cases the action of the well-indicated remedy does not improve the case permanently, even though the potency be raised. There is a barrier, a resistance to the remedy working as it should. This "wall", as Burnett would call it, is an underlying layer deep within the constitution, and probably the inherited cause of disease which is capable of manifesting itself in a variety of ways. We understand this more fully when we realise that disease is a condition and not an entity. The importance of the nosodes in the breaking down of these walls which we so often come up against in patients, cannot be over emphasised. The tubercular miasm/diathesis/dyscrasia, call it what you will, is a very real barrier to the action of a "well-selected" remedy. You will see from the notes the large number of our major polychrests which are linked with the tubercular diathesis. When you have a good response from a remedy and then find that neither repetition nor increasing the potency has the desired effect do not desert the remedy to look for another. Consider the symptoms of the nosodes in the case and after administering the appropriate one you will find that your original remedy is still indicated and will now progress the case.

Hahnemann in the organon §173,175,176,215 refers to the "one sided cases". Kent in his Materia Medica under Magnesium carbonicum writes, "the cases that are hard to manage and difficult to find remedies for - they fit into the lingering state of tuberculosis - their trouble is so latent their symptoms do not come out. They are the one-sided cases spoken of by Hahnemann".

Most of the writers to which we normally refer give the miasm psora, pseudo-psora, sycosis and syphilis but not tubercular as such. The only books I know of which contain substantial references to Tuberculinum and Bacillinum are: HC Allen's Materia Medica of the Nosodes in which he refers to both, Burnett's works (Bacillinum), JH Clarke's Dictionary of Practical Materia Medica (Tuberculinum and Bacillinum), Roberts' Principles and Art of Cure by Homœopathy where he refers to tuberculosis under the syphilitic stigma and Kent's Materia Medica on Tuberculinum. In JH Allen's 'The Chronic Miasms' p23, he does not leave us completely clear as to what he meant by pseudo-psora and we can only surmise a reference to tubercular. More recent additions to knowledge have been predominantly French and these are given in the notes.

Schmidt preferred to use Tuberculinum bovinum. He also disagreed that tuberculosis is psora - syphilis, for he considered it to be psora - sycosis.
Nebel Montreux of Switzerland regarded tuberculosis as synonymous with psora.
Dr Vannier of France subdivided psora into a combination of tuberculosis and psora.

Quoting from Roberts under the syphilitic stigma he remarks, "Tuberculosis does not comprise the established tuberculous lesion such as those of the lungs, glands, bones, but there is a preceding stage which the French call 'etat tuberculinique', meaning tuberculinism, where there is no tubercle bacillus."

It is Grimmer who considered cancerous states to be built on the tubercular diathesis. In these cases, the stethoscope or tests give little help in finding the reasons for tired languid conditions.

A useful method of picking up on the nosodes in a case is to make a special note whenever they appear in your repertorisation. This means that having selected your rubrics and begun your elimination you should note down in the margin any nosodes which appear in any of the rubrics you look at. The same rule should be applied to Thuja. In this way you have an idea of the possible blocks in the case and you can be at the ready if they come to the fore.

As Wright Hubbard comments, symptoms are often hard to find in infants and the young, the giving of the correct nosode will bring out the chronic symptoms for further prescribing. Her picture of tuber-cular children is:

> Those with violent tempers, tantrums, kicking
> and scratching screaming on the floor.
> Angel faced infant.
> Alabaster skin.
> No perseverance or concentration.
> Tendency to frequent coughs and colds.
> Listless, weak, glandular troubles.

She comments that Bacillinum is more suited in actual cases of tuberculosis or where there is a secondary infection and that Tuberculinum should rather be used where there is an inherited ten-dency to the disease. If several nosodes are indicated from the family stream then we must be guided to our first choice by the eval-uated symptoms of the case. When that layer is cleared away the underlying miasm will then become uppermost.

You will find that Tuberculinum is often indicated in the various stages of life. Childhood and adolescence are obvious times of growth and change when the tubercular picture comes to the fore. Similarly the tubercular state may well be precipitated in the years of maturity by emotional or environmental stresses and as old age pro-gresses so the latent psoric-syphilitic state can again manifest itself.

"No practice in homœopathy can develop its best results without the use of Tuberculinum and Bacillinum."

- 3 -
Case Examples

Case 1   Child with constant coughing from yet another cold. Capricious, difficult to please, gets epistaxis and frequently responds well to Ipecac.

Tuberculinum will prevent these recurrences. However the child is only well for a short time after the Tub and now has a persistent symptom of not being able to sleep, being unable to wake in the morning and having developed an itch and soreness to the anus. A fissure is in evidence. There are no other symptoms for a particular remedy but the nightly aggravation, weakness in the morning, fissure and the short improvement under Tuberculinum means we must now look to Syphilinum.

In cases such as this the family history will reveal conditions like cancer, hayfever, chilblains, heart disease, alcoholism, mental illness, etc.

Case 2   Female 32 years old. Tall, dark and depressed.

Head - feeling of compression. Wakes up with a sense of tightness which lasts the whole day. Feels her scalp is tight.

Tub   She presses it for relief. This day after day makes her weak.

Tub   Hair is lustreless and has a tendency to fall out.

Tub   Breasts swell before menses, most painful.

Stomach feels bloated and tight with constriction. Gradual feeling that she cannot eat anymore as the area of the pyloric goes into spasm and remains tight.

Tub   Rectum also feels sense of constriction. Stools pass with such difficulty, has to strain with little result.

Haemorrhoids uncomfortable and full, not painful.

Menses. Copious, dark to black, clotted with bearing down and heaviness. Excessive pruritis of the vulva. This means she has aversion to sex. Suffers from vaginismus.

Extremities feel constricted with the same kind of tightness - hips, thighs, knees, feet.

Tub   General.   < Sitting - gets restless.
                   < Open air and sunshine.

Tub   Mentals. Constant changing moods. Goes from extremes of tempers - gaiety to depressions. Restless. Gets really annoyed with fools, won't suffer them at all - let alone lightly. Isolates herself as a result of this attitude. Feels alone and goes off on her own.

The Essence of the Case:

Spasms. Tightness. Constrictions in all parts of the body. Restless.
Changeable moods. Critical. Contemptuous.
Constipation - ineffectual urging.
Menses black.

Repertorisation from Kent's Repertory:

Genitalia, female, metrorrhagia, black : p729.
Generalities, constriction internally : p1351.
Mind, censorious : p10.
Mind, contemptuous : p16.
Mind, mood, changeable : p68.
Rectum, constipation, ineffectual urging and straining : p607.
Exty, tension, (hip, thigh, knee, feet), < sitting : pp1204-1206.
Head, contraction of scalp, sensation of : p114.
Head, constriction : p112.

Remedy given:

Platina 1M, one dose.

The follow ups:

The constipation cleared.
Sensation of tightness much improved in all areas.
Headaches generally diminished.

Two months later there was a return of headache tension and constriction, not quite as intense, but she was fearful they would be.

Because of the underlying Tuberculinum of the case, confirmed by
the childhood ailments of continual sore throats, epistaxis, temper
tantrums and ringworm, it was now clear that Tuberculinum bovinum was needed to make the case permanently cured.

The second choice may have been to go higher in the Platina but all
the other symptoms had improved under Platina 1M and the slipping
of the head tensions and weakness, A.M. on waking, is a characteristic Tuberculinum symptom. Platina may still be needed later but at
this stage it could not hold.

Tuberculinum bovinum 200 [3] much improved the case for about 6
months. When the symptom of the head tightness returned slightly
again, Tuberculinum bovinum 1M completed the case. No further
remedies were given.

There are obviously variations according to individual response.

If for example, in case 2 the patient had still demonstrated a pre-
dominance of Platina symptoms then, heeding the uppermost

3. C potency throughout unless otherwise stated.

indications, a higher potency of Platina would have been appropriate. If that higher potency had been disappointing then we would
have known that Platina could have done little more because of the
underlying tubercular miasm. Tuberculinum would therefore be
needed.

Should the Tuberculinum only hold for a limited time and the
Platina symptoms again return then the Platina must be repeated in
the same potency as before. It will be found that this time it will be
more effective because Tuberculinum has removed the barrier.

"Never desert the remedy which has been of most help"

It is necessary here to remember Burnett's invaluable injunction that
Bacillinum or Tuberculinum may not even act until Thuja has been
given, when indicated. This is to remove the vaccination or sycotic
barrier.

- 4 -
Tuberculinum in Psycho-Pathology - Barbancy 1976

The following information is from a paper by Barbancy (Bordeaux, France, 1976) who is a psychiatrist. The combination of psychiatric terms together with difficulty in finding an exact English translation for certain words leads to some rather awkward phraseology. Nevertheless the picture she paints of mental and emotional turmoil in the tubercular type is still a masterpiece.

"A disease of society"
"A horrid metastasis of civilisation"

Behaviours not socially adapted.

Troubles of psychic sphere or secondary effects after classical therapeutics (fat, flabby and slack).

Lack of self-defence.

Somatic and psychological aggressions.

Congenital difficulties to live and survive.

1)   *Fatigue* - always latent - alternates with euphoric activity or hyper-excitability.
Can isolate themselves in a pathological seclusion.

2) *Vulnerable* - physically and mentally.

Alternating States

Studious enthusiasm	Progressive loss of interest
Trust	Doubt
Exaltation	Indifference
Efficacious days of study	Total incapacity to work
Creative inspiration	Long periods of sterility
Vivid and precise	Lost in a fog out of which it is difficult to come
Menaced - as if threatened by themselves and the outside world - and enthusiastic	Painful to continue to take interest, to stand fast, to hold conversation
Lovers of beauty, harmony, idealism - dream world	Realisation of mental degradation is atrocious

3) *Level of effectivity*

Intense need of certitude and security (Puls)	Concerned with independence (Nat mur, Phos)

All disharmony in his environment hurts him, all frustration of affections real or felt as such can be a source of depression. One can blame teachers and educational failings or rant at the state of society, but there is the inescapable fact of a "fragile being".

Behaviour is sometimes soft and fraternal	Grumpy and solitary, eruptions of violence, aggression, defence
Generosity	Vindictiveness
Loves the absolute, idealistic in moral spheres, harmony and beauty	Cynical

These contradictions express themselves as the need
to change - travellers without frontiers, unceasing
projects, new jobs - the desire to change ones life
even to abandoning family, studies and comfort -
always hoping to be better elsewhere.

All this leads to physical collapse, nervous depression or a thera-
peutic rectification and the rebuilding of the personality. The "flow"
will reveal itself any time under shock, illness, mourning, loss of
security and affections and passes onto:

Organic symptoms   -   TB - larynx, pulmonary
                   -   Psychosomatic illness

It is important that they posses either creative capacity or artistic
aptitude - literary, musical, graphic. Expressing originality in spite
of dangers from artificial stimulation by alcohol or drugs.
As long as the need to create exists then equilibrium remains possible, otherwise suicide is a constant temptation.

Psycho-Pathology in:

1)   **Childhood** is relatively rare.
     Children need physical treatment (Sil), although constant ill-
     ness and therefore solitude may turn them to dreamers full of
     imagination. Others are unstable, agitated, hyperactive,
     opposing and violent, having a phobia to being touched -
     desiring it or averse to it (even by the mother). Untreatable in
     medical examinations - screaming and kicking such that you
     can't get near them.

2)   **Adolescent crisis.**
     Characterised by variability of moods - excitability, modifi-
     cations of thoughts and affections.
     a) Reactions excessive to exterior influences (Iodum,
        Spongia).

b) Psychic upsets and difficulties of integration, infantile regression to avoid problems of sexuality (Sil, Abrot, Sanic).

c) Phobia syndromes, eg. non acceptance of body - "I'm ugly", leading to self mutilating conduct, self destructive (Kali brom, Nat mur, Phos, Staph).

3) ***Schizophrenic syndrome.***
  - Hebephrenic is gravest form.
  - Failure in evolution towards maturity.
  - Indifference in the affections (Sep).
  - Isolation and dreaming (frequent in adolescents).
  - Means to obtain attention.
  - Concentration and memory collapse.
  - Escape from the constraints of reality.
  - Despair of not being able to adjust to reality.
  - Believe all around are alien - on the borders of insanity.
  - Oddities of speech and disassociation of thought - stereotyped patterns of speech are mechanisms of defence against the phobias.
  - Vacillate between tenacious withdrawal or crying out for help indirectly or symbolically, eg. attempted suicide.

In any of these three situations we should rather use an indicated remedy other than Tuberculinum in case of aggravation. Tuberculinum will be necessary if the indicated remedies do not work.

The numerous states of mental weakness and imbalance which we see in such remedies as Ignatia, Natrum carbonicum, Sepia and Lycopodium will only be properly stabilised by the use of Tuberculinum in these cases.

From all of the above we can see that Tuberculinum is a very important remedy in anxiety neuroses of the schizoid type and neurotic asthenics. Similarly in the confusional states of those growing old in patients whose remedies are Silica, Arsenicum or Iodum.

- 4 -
Bacillinum

Burnetts proving in 1892 used bacilli tubercles from human lung tissue.

Burnett's many little booklets ('Delicate, Backward, Puny and Stunted Children' and 'Curability of Tumours' etc.) are a joy to read and the following data has been drawn from them.

< Night, early A.M., cold air.   Complementary remedies are Calc-c, Calc-p, Phos, Kali-c, Psorinum.

The tubercular diathesis or active TB are favourably influenced by this nosode - however only non-complicated cases and not too advanced TB. (Psorinum is needed in advanced cases).

Respiratory:

Congestion of the lungs and catarrh of such.
Oppression, coarse bubbling rales, purulent expectoration.
Chronic cough with concomitants of heat and sweat at night.
Wheezing - dyspnœa with suffocative attacks at night.
Old people with chronic catarrhal symptoms and feeble pulmonary circulation.
Throat studded with tubercles, feverish, expectorates blood and pus.
Aphonia.
Phlegm < A.M.

Indurated Glands:

Tubercular enlargement of the cervical and mesenteric lymph nodes.

Look for strumous scar on the neck of the patient indicating removal of tubercular glands.

Groin full of small indurated glands.

Skin Conditions:

Ringworm.

Ulcerative eruptions of the nose.

Urticaria, "bat-wing" discolouration of nose/cheek junction.

Alopecia or bald patches of the head, beard, moustache.

Acne - symbolises the "dash" of TB that lurks behind (if pustular and scarring use vaccinium or variolinum).

Eczematous (redness of eyelid margin).

Brownish spots/blotches on face.

Clinical:

Rheumatoid arthritis - may be followed by Thuja or Psorinum.

Headaches - long lasting pains in the head - tubercular meningitis.

Menorrhagia.

Pelvic TB - you may need Hydrastis tincture to follow.

Insomnia.

Cancer of pylorus. (Burnett says weekly dose).

Tubercles on head.

String of little nuts (tubercles) on wrists, knees, ankles, neck.

< Touch.

Activities of joints restricted by the colonies of tubercles.

Strawberry tongue.

Rachitis - curvature of the spine.

Clammy hands and feet (cold) - night sweats.

Cretinous idiots.

Epistaxis.

Provings:

1) Pain in glands of neck (submaxillary, cervical), < turning head, < right side.
2) Pains deep in the head.
3) Aching in the teeth, especially lower, < cold air.
4) Sharp pains of short duration in chest and various parts of the body.
5) Pain left knee < walking, > walking.
6) Nasal catarrh, pricking in throat or larynx, sudden cough <A.M. rising, < night. Easy expectoration. Sharp pain in chest through to left scapula > warmth.
7) Indolent pimples - will not heal.
8) Dusky tawny skin - tans easily without going red.

If TB from cancerous parentage Bacillinum alone will not suffice.

Sometimes Bacillinum will not act until Thuja has been given - it is thought to remove the vaccination or sycotic layer.

Other References to Bacillinum

H.C.Allen:

When Burnett feared that TB was around he never went below 200.
Doses can be administered every 6-10 days (Burnett's practice).
At certain stages of TB, Bacillinum ceases to act curatively (once past acute) and then Psorinum is needed for the chronic state.
Bacillinum is rapid in its action - will work within hours.
One or two doses a week will relieve TB cough, night sweats and fever even though it doesn't cure advanced TB.
Useful in alcoholism, syphilis, malaria, anaemia, vaccinosis, sclerosis.
Generally it relieves congestion of lungs, coughs and night sweats whether tubercular or not.

Long:

Pneumonia - "the first remedy I think of is Bacillinum unless there are ample indications for another - it seems to finish the case".
Better in acute lung conditions and Tuberculinum Koch in chronic.

J.H.Clarke:

Mentally taciturn, sulky, snappish, irritable, morose, depressed, melancholic, whining, complaining.
Drum belly, tabes mesenterica, indurated inguinals, diarrhoea, windy dyspepsia.
Grinds teeth in sleep.
Green discoloured teeth.
Headaches - hoop/band sensation, pains deep in < motion.

W.Boericke:

Tendency to take cold.
Sudden diarrhoea before breakfast.
Early stages of tubercular glands, joints, skin, bones.

Cartier:

In acute conditions Bacillinum can be used 4 hourly.
Body lice (pthiriasis).

Wining:

For the 1914/18 flu - the remedy that prevented the collapse.

Anshutz:

Sputum is less abundant, less purulent, less green, more aerated.
Pseudo-phymic bronchitis - a complication often found with
influenza and mistaken for TB. (Even if the bacillus of TB is present! Often people possess tuberculous lesions). Koch's bacillus
found in nasal secretions of hospital nurses.

Different types as:
Pseudo-tuberculosis.
Zoogleic-tuberculosis.
Pseudo-bacillosis of bovine origin.
Pseudo-bacillosis of a strepto-bacillar origin.
Professional tuberculosis - those exposed to breathe fumes.

Bacillinum is a powerful moderator of the muco-purulent secretion
of TB.

Published cases for: Acute bronchitis.
                                 Influenza.
                                 Diarrhoeas.
                                 Syphilitic eruptions.
                                 Cystitis.
                                 Ringworm of the scalp.
                                 Nephritis.
                                 Idiocy - cretinism.
                                 Retarded dentition.
                                 Gout. Rheumatism.

Characteristics for non-tuberculous diseases of the respiratory organs. Two important ones are:
1) Oppression
2) Muco-purulent expectoration.

Dyspnoea resulting from bronchial and pulmonary obstruction caused by a super abundance of secretion is marvelously relieved by Bacillinum.

Mersch:

Oppression in pulmonary catarrh, where dyspnoea is a characteristic symptom and is more distressing than the cough.

Bronchial asthma - In aged, from colds, which go to obstruction of the bronchial tubes. Has to sit up. Struggling to breathe in. Phos or Ars in 30 potency at long intervals.

Asthma - Incessant cough, yellow putrid mucus, thick, opaque, sleepless nights.

Chronic catarrhs - dyspnoea - difficulty in coughing - suffocation nights.
Pulmonary congestions after colds.
Acute cases: Bacillinum 30 every 3 days.

Chronic cases: Bacillinum 30, 100, 200 every week to 2 weeks.

Tuberculinum Aviare - in influenzal bronchitis.
Expectoration thick putrid sputa.
Influenzal coughs - invasion sudden and severe.
It relieves the debility. Improves appetite.
Considerable coughs. Little dyspnoea (opposite to Bacillinum).
Acute inflammatory extremely irritating cough.
Cough fatigues.

Comparison of Bacillinum and Tuberculinum

Bacillinum

Pneumonia
> In acute lung conditions. Cough < rising.
Loosens cough Phlegm < A.M.
Chronic cough & heat & sweats night
    Wheezing   Expect. (Spong)
      NIGHT Bubbly, briny.
    Dyspnoea   Purulent pus

Short sharp pains chest to left scapula.
Tendency for colds - flu's respiratory
Enlargement of glands with pains.
Cervical < turning head to side. Right.
String of nuts - (tubercles) wrists, knees, ankles, neck
                      < touch

Deep in headaches - long lasting. Tubercular.
Meningitis. Hoop. Band. < Motion.
Strawberry tongue.
Epistaxis.
Catarrhs - prickings larynx, throat.(Cedr, Tell, Verat,
Chronic catarrhs in aged.   Calc-f, Lach, Manc)
Skin tans easily - tawny colour.
Acne (pustular: Vaccinum, Variolinum).
Eczematous redness of eyelids.
Brownish blotches - bat-wing across nose/cheeks.
Pimples won't heal.
Alopecia - head, beard, moustache.
Green discoloured teeth.

Tuberculinum

Dry hacking cough.
> In chronic lung conditions.

Rumex type coughs < open air.
Night sweats.
Broncho-pneumonia in children. Dyspnoea.
Croup. Thick yellow expectoration. Green expectoration
(Puls, Stann , Psor, Kali-c).
Tendency for colds. Influenzas.
Recurrent sore throats (Psor, Syph). Enlarged tonsils.
Glands goitre.

Chronic sick headaches. Menstrual headaches.
As if would burst.

Adenoids. Hayfever.

> Stove heat. Eczema.
Acne. Dermatitis.
Susceptibility to Rhus tox poisonings. Itching all over body
> rubbing.
Rash - abdomen and back - red to brownish, as if secondary
syphilis.
Alopecia. Tinea barbae.
Teething in babes - swollen gums (Calc, Bell).

Body lice. Ringworm.
Drum belly (Tabes mesenterica)
    Indurated inguinals.
    Diarrhoea.
    Windy dyspepsia.
    Sudden diarrhoea before breakfast.

Head lice.

Excoriation rectum. Morning diarrhoeas.
Haemorrhage of the bowels.
Fistula of anus (Psoric-Tubercular).
Constipation. Bleeding haemorrhoids.
Liver upsets tendency.
Emaciation with great appetite.
Family history of TB.

Consumptives.
Old people - when chronic conditions not well marked.
Shortens convalescence.
Rheumatoid arthritis. (Tub res) Thuja, Psorinum.
Rachitis. Curvature of spine.

Osteoporosis. Decalcification.
Wens of knee, wrist, head, with excessive fluid.
< Motion in severe joint pains.
Acute articular rheumatism.
Callosities of feet. Ingrown toenails.
Night sweats. Intermittent fever.
Heat with sweats.
Flushings and burnings of heat.

Joints - (Follow by Thuja, Psor.)

Hands and feet cold and clammy - Night sweats.

Frequent dental cases.

Insomnia.
Grinds teeth at night.
Teeth ache < cold air.
Cretins.

Backward children.
Epilepsy.

Cancer of pyloris (Weekly dose - Burnett).

Menorrhagia (copious).

Mentally taciturn. Sulky. Irritable.
Morose. Depressed. Complainers.
Melancholic.

< AM = phlegm.
< Nights
< Early AM.
< Cold air.

Complementaries:
Calc, Calc-p, Phos, Kali-c, Psor.

Amenorrhoea. Late menses (Puls).
Repeated miscarriages. Dysmenorrhoea.
Bright's disease.
Fears dogs, cats.   < Waking. Tired.
Apprehension. Worries over trifles.
Depressed. Weepy. Melancholic.
Negative.   < Damp weather.
Insanity. Won't talk, no incentive.
Extrovert. Restless - mind especially.
Obstinate. Contrary. Peevish when ill.
Excuses not to work - exhaustion.
Look younger than they are.
Critical. Selfish.
Wants to rush - breaks things results in > tensions.
Tremors. Odd behaviour.
Sexual troubles of young boys; erections early.
< AM.   > Frosty crisp air.
< Cold.   > Warm bed, rest.
< Damp weather.   > Delicacies
< Standing.   sweets & smoked
                         meats.
< After pregnancy (depressed)> Pregnancy.
< Short walks (fatigue).   > Day before (Psor).
Complementaries:
Rhus, Bell, Calc, Calc-p, Lach, Kali-c, Nat-m, Phos,
Sil, Sulph, Chin, Dros, Puls, Sul-i, Ars-i, Psor.

- 8 -
Tuberculinum

E. Long:

Taken from the case note book of E.Long (out of print) which belonged to Noel Puddephatt who taught George Vithoulkas and myself.

While there is undoubtedly great similarity in the pathogenetic sphere of the various Tuberculinums, I feel confident that there is a difference, and that it would amply repay a most careful and complete research. In the more brilliant results obtained with any of our remedies the finer selection relies on the distinctions. In a rough way I find...

Bacillinum	Is better suited to acute manifestations of lung troubles.
Tub Koch	Is better suited to chronic results of pneumonia.
Bacillinum	Is the first remedy I think of in pneumonia unless there are ample indications for another. Even if another remedy leads in the acute turmoil, I find that Bacillinum is needed to finish the attack. The cough loosens, the pain subsides and the lungs are freed from the accumulation.
	In old people it acts like a charm. It is not a specific remedy for every case, but in those cases where the indications are not well marked, and as a finisher to the case, it shortens convalescence time. (You may need its complementary, Psorinum. - Creasy.).

In general consumptive conditions I have had good results, quick and satisfactory. I'm sure Tub would do, but because of the good results obtained I prefer Bacillinum in these cases.

Tub bov   Incipient stages of hip joint disease, Tuberculinum has promptly relieved.

Tub aviare   For poorly treated influenza, especially when the lungs are involved.

Tub Koch   Think of more in tubercular conditions of the skin.

There is evidently a friendly and complementary relationship between Calcarea carbonica and Tuberculinum. Psorinum also has this close relationship to Tuberculinum. In any lack of reaction to the well indicated remedy it often comes in to arouse the vital energies of these weak cases.

As a general rule the nosodes are the best for nondescript and obscure cases. They will generally clear the cobwebs from the case leading to the curative remedy, and might even be the curative remedy in the chronic form of disease.

Repetition of Tuberculinum:
My plan, adopted after a long experience of its use in chronic cases, is to select a medium potency upwards, give 2 to 3 doses twelve hours apart and then to repeat according to the need in the progress of the case. Intervals, if necessary, of up to 28 days. Waiting on the action of the remedy is not merely that there should be some action, but as Hahnemann expresses it, "a strikingly increasing amelioration". Waiting for 40 to 100 days is more the exception than the rule.

You will notice that the most frequently indicated remedies needing Tuberculinum to complete the case are:
Bell, Calc-c, Calc-p, Lach, Kali-c, Nat-m, Phos, Sil, Sulph, China, Dros, Puls, Sulph-i, Ars-i, Psor.

Obtained from Clarke - I have found that in women who have had hydrocephalic children who have died, there is a TB basis. If pregnant again a number of doses of Sulphur 6 to be followed by Calc-phos 6 should be administered throughout the pregnancy.

Nebel Montreux. (From Hom. World 1904):

Chronic sick headaches - even to helping patients dispense with glasses.
Constipation and bleeding haemorrhoids.
Intermittent fever, returning annually, has always a psoric or TB diathesis.
Bright's disease is generally tubercular.
We rarely have a case of insanity without an inherited psoric or TB diathesis.
Typhoid always occurs in psoric or tubercular patients.
In pneumonia, after the aconite stage has passed and hepatisation takes place, in almost 9 out of 10 cases the remedy needed is apt to be Sulphur or Iodum - these correspond to the psoric constitution of the patient. If a few members of the family have had pneumonia or TB then Sulphur will not be deep enough and it will require Tuberculinum to completely cure the patient. I have applied this suggestion in more conditions than pneumonia with splendid results.

Influenza - generally from January to March in the TB type.
Teething in babies. If Belladonna is indicated in the swollen gums with lots of pain, then Calc is the chronic. But if there are meningeal troubles you will need Tuberculinum.
Menstrual headaches of intensity often need Tuberculinum or Psorinum.
Dysmenorrhoea and hysteria are always tubercular.
Nocturnal enuresis - Tuberculinum will cure a third of these cases.
Coughs. In Rumex type coughs which are worse in the open air, where they must cover the mouth and nostrils to prevent the cough, if the cough is apt to return on the next exposure to cold then Tuberculinum will be needed to cure.
Fistula of the anus is always a tubercular or psoric diathesis.

Carcinoma and sarcoma have all the miasms behind them.

Wens of the wrist and excess synovial fluid of the knee often call for Calcarea or Tuberculinum. Susceptibility to poisoning by Rhus tox is of a tubercular diathesis. They have a weakened vitality for their powers of resistance are poor. You may cure your patients for a time but in the majority of cases you will need to use Tuberculinum to prevent recurrences. This hint led me to prove that Rhus and Tuberculinum are complementary.

You will never find a drunkard except in a miasmatic patient and similarly ingrowing toenails and callosites on the soles of the feet show a psoric and tubercular diathesis.

Croup, asthma, hay fever, ringworm, Bright's disease, haemorrhage of the bowels and goitre are always of a tubercular diathesis.

Belladonna, Tuberculinum and Natrum muriaticum are often a complementary trio.

"In active TB (consumption) do not give Phosphorus, Sulphur, Psorinum, Silica, Sulphuric acid, Acetic acid or even a metal, but, use a vegetable remedy or Tuberculinum and hand them down to the grave in peace".

Priestman:

Downy hair on face and back.
Silky hair.
Long lashes.
Good complexion.
Pale pink scurf patches on face.
Apprehension.
Fear of animals, especially dogs.
Worries over trifles.
Sensitive to cold and damp.
Depressed, weepy, melancholic and hopeless in damp weather.
Thrives in frosty, crisp air.

Very energetic to a certain point then reaches a sudden draining of strength and then needs to lie down to rest.

Irritability and loss of appetite.

Critical and censorious - selfish.

Peevish, easily upset when ill.

Anger and sudden uncontrollable passion followed by weakness and exhaustion in good natured people.

Can't be bothered - will not talk or be talked to.

Intense restlessness of body but especially the mind.

Craves change of occupation or surroundings - desires to travel.

Sensitive to all impressions and the needs of others.

Reckless and then over-remorseful.

Stupor (eg. after insomnia).

Breaks things, rushes around to relieve nervous tension.

Drowsy and can't sleep, dreams vividly, unrefreshing sleep.

Tendency to colds, coughs, bronchitis.

Headaches as if the head would burst and of long lasting duration.

< Standing.	> Rest.
< Over fatigue.	> During pregnancy.
< After pregnancy.	

Pulford:

Leading remedy for red face in afternoon.

Leading remedy for weakness from night sweats.

Dullness of mind.

Epistaxis.

Circumscribed cheeks - or pale sickly face.

Heat of face.

Desires delicacies and smoked meat.

Cough dry and hacking.

Expectoration thick and yellow.

Oppression of chest.

Heat with sweat.

Tendency to take cold.

Weariness > warm bed.

Glandular enlargements.

Obstinate, contrary.

Negativism - can only say no.

Extrovert.

Cosmopolitan.

Likes excess of everything except work which exhausts.

Look younger than they are.

Family history of TB, asthma, migraine, dermatitis, arthritis, behavioural disorders, chronic dysmenorrhoea.

Sananes:

Bad childhood illnesses - whooping cough, bronchitis, measles, pleurisy, rhinopharyngitis. Febrile episodes of two or three days without cause.

Amenorrhoea. Late menses (Pulsatilla). Repeated miscarriages.

Hypersensitive to pain.

Peripheral congestion.

Mucus problems. Swellings of all the glands.

< Diarrhoea, vomiting, perspiration.

> Air.

Osteoporosis. Decalcification. Dehydration. (Calc-p, Nat-m, Sil).

Sensitive to cold.

Constipation. Tendency to liver upsets.

Abnormal hunger before headaches (Psor, Phos).

Abnormal hunger but never gains weight.

Abnormal growth where linked with other tubercular aspects.

Dermatitis. Purulent cutaneous attacks. Acne (Dulc, Merc, Hepar).

Burning, areas and generally (Sulph).

Exhausted in respiratory troubles and too weak to speak (Stann).

Diarrhoea alternating with constipation.

Feet cold with fever.

> Before an aggravation; well the day before (Psor).

Four 'swords' of Tuberculinum	Acutes of Tuberculinum
• Calcarea phosphorica • Drosera • Natrum muriaticum • Silica	• Ferrum phosphorica • Sulphur iodum finishes off the case

Use Tuberculinum Koch (rather than Tuberculinum bovinum) where perspiration predominates and similarly Tuberculinum residium if sinus predominates.

Schlegel:

Irritability on waking A.M.,add Tuberculinum to Kent p.60
Weeping from music. Add Ambr, Lyc, Nat-m, Phos, Ph-ac, Tarent, Tub, Thuja, Sep. to Kent p.94.
Adenoids.
Recurrent sore throats.
Sexual troubles especially in young boys, excessive.
Change of weather aggravates.
Chronic cystitis.
Kidney disease (Bright's).
Tuberculosis (Use high potencies).
Tendency for colds.
Backward children.
Enlarged tonsils.
Skin affections.
Acute articular rheumatism.
Very sensitive mentally and physically.
Tremors.
Epilepsy.
Patient is odd.
Benign breast tumours.
Dysmenorrhoea.
Broncho-pneumonia in children.
Frequent repetition is necessary in childhood diseases.

Other Preparations of Tuberculinum

Tuberculinum aviare (Proving by F.E.Boericke and Taffel).
References by Boer, Jousset and Wheeler.

Tuberculinum aviare has a more gentle action than Tuberculinum bovinum or Koch. It can be used in acute or sub-acute febrile periods. Diminishes incessant tickling cough - acute or chronic.
Acutes which may develop into bronchial pneumonia. Any pulmonary affections with profuse expectoration, potency 100 or 200 - can be repeated 24/48 hours.
Influenzinal bronchitis, especially if remedies are slipping all the time.
It is useful where there is no vital reaction to the indicated acute remedy. The person is low (Psorinum).
Especially indicated in otitis when states refuse to clear up.
Itching of palms of hands and ears.
Improves appetite if lost.

Tuberculinum residium (Provings by Sananes and Horveilleur).

Sycotic.
Fibrositis.
Rheumatic complaints.
Finger contractions (Duployen) (Causticum, Thuja).
A fat Natrum muriaticum could be Tub-r (Dr Sananes).
Stiffness of forearms - persistent writer's cramp.
(Mag phos, Cuprum, Cimicifuga, Causticum).
Sinus predominates.

Bacillinum Testium

W.Boericke - Acts especially on lower half of body.
Burnett - Undescended testicle.

- 10 -
Rubrics Containing Tuberculinum

All rubrics are from Kent's repertory unless otherwise stated. The mind section is complete with rubrics from the reputable authors (in brackets). The other sections are largely made up of the characteristics of Tuberculinum.

Mind:

Abstraction of mind (Schmidt)
Abusive
Ailments from, excitement, emotional (Schmidt)
Ailments from, work, mental (Schmidt)
Anger, irascibility (Boger)
Anger, throws things away (Schmidt)
Anger, waking on (Schmidt)
Answers 'NO' to all questions (Schmidt)
Anticipation, dentist, physician, before going to (Schmidt)
Anxiety, evening (Kent)
Anxiety, children in (Schmidt)
Anxiety, midnight before (Kent)
Anxiety - fever, during
Anxiety, headache with
Break things, desire to
Change, desire for (Kent, Boger, Schmidt)
Cheerful, gay, mirthful
Confusion of mind (Boger)
Confusion, walking, while, air, in open
Cursing
Delerium (Knerr)
Delusions (Knerr)
Delusions, large, people seem too (during vertigo) (Schmidt)
Delusions, snakes in and around her (Boger)
Dclusions, strange, familiar things seem (Schmidt)
Despair
Destructiveness
Dipsomania, alcoholism (Boericke)

Dullness - sluggishness

Dullness, children in (Schmidt)

Escape, attempts to

Excitement, excitable

Exertion, agg. from mental (Schmidt)

Fear, apprehension, dread (Boger)

Fear, animals, of (Boger, Schmidt)

Fear, dogs, of

Fear, happen, something will

Fear, waking on (Boger, Schmidt)

Forgetful

Heedless (Boger)*Hopeful*

Ideas, abundant, clearness of mind

Idiocy

Impulse, run, to (Schmidt)

Indifference, apathy (Boger, Schmidt)

Indolence, aversion to work (Schmidt)

Industrious, mania for work (Schmidt)

Insanity, madness (Kent, Schmidt)

Insanity, madness, alternating mental with physical symptoms (Kent)

Insanity, madness, travel, with desire to (Kent)

Irritability

Irritability, morning, waking on (Schmidt)

Irritability, children, in (Schmidt)

Irritability, waking on (Schmidt)

Looked at, cannot bear to be (Schmidt)

Loquacity, changing quickly from one subject to another (Boger)

Loquacity - heat, during

Mania (Clarke)

Memory - weakness of

Mental symptoms alternating with physical (Kent)

Moaning, groaning, whining (Knerr, Schmidt)

Mood - alternating

Mood - changeable, variable

Music amel. (Boger, Schmidt)

Obstinate, headstrong (Boger, Schmidt)

Obstinate, headstrong, children (Schmidt)

Offended easily, takes everything in bad part (Schmidt)

Pull ones hair, desire to (Schmidt)

Quarrelsome, scolding (Schmidt)

Restlessness (Schmidt)

Restlessness, night (Kent)

Restlessness, children, in (Schmidt)

Sadness, despondency, dejection, mental depression, gloom, melancholy (Boger, Schmidt, Boericke)

Sensitive, oversensitive (Boger)

Sensitive, oversensitive, noise to (Schmidt)

Shrieking

Shrieking, children in (Schmidt)

Shrieking, children in, sleep, during (Knerr)

Shrieking, sleep, during (Kent, Knerr, Schmidt, Boericke)

Speech - nonsense

Starting, startled (Boericke)

Starts - sleep, on falling

Strange - everything seems

Striking himself, knocking his head against wall and things (Schmidt)

Suicidal disposition (Boger)

Talk, indisposed to, desire to be silent, taciturn (Kent)

Talk, sleep in (Kent)

Thoughts - persistent

Thoughts - persistent, night

Thoughts, tormenting, night (Kent)

Threatening (Schmidt)

Throws things away (Boger)

Throws things, persons, at (Schmidt)

Torments himself (Boger)

Travel - desire to

Trifles seem important (Boger)

Wanders, desire to (Schmidt)

Weary of life (Kent)

Weeping, spoken to, when (Knerr)

Work, aversion to mental

Head:

Bores, head in pillow
Inflammation of brain, tubercular
Motions, rolling head
Pain, periodic headache
Pain, periodic, every seven days
Pain, periodic, every fourteen days
Pain, reading <
Pain, straining eyes, from

Eye:

Astigmatism
Eruptions lids, scaly herpes, margins
Eruptions, lids, scurfy (Schmidt)
Pain - sore, (bruised, tender)
Pain - sore, moving eyes
Pain - turning sideways
Photophobia
Pupils, contracted
Pupils - insensible to light
Stabismus

Vision:

Colours - blue
Colours - green
Colours - halo of, around light
Hemiopia - horizontal
Images too long rtained
Myopia
Run - together, letters

Ear:

Discharges - offensive
Discharges - purulent

Noises - in
Noises in, right
Noises, chirping
Pain
Pain - night
Pain, waking on
Stopped sensation
Stopped sensation, right

Hearing:

Acute - to noises

Nose:

Catarrh
Coryza - chronic, long continued
Coryza, nose cold
Discharge - bloody
Discharge - copious
Discharge - crusts, scabs, inside
Discharge - offensive, foetid, cheese like
Discharge - posterior nares (see catarrh)
Discharge - purulent
Discharge - thick
Discharge - yellow
Epistaxis
Epistaxis - blood, bright
Epistaxis - blood, clotted
Itching
Pain - sore inside
Perspiration on
Swelling

Face:

Discoloured - blue, during chill
Discoloured - pale

Discoloured - red, afternoon
Discoloured - red, circumscribed
Discoloured - red, during chill
Discoloured - red during fever
Discoloured - red, lips
Discoloured - sickly colour
Discoloured - yellow, intermittent,in
Eruptions - acne
Eruptions - acne rosacea
Eruptions - comedones
Eruptions - comedones, ulcerating
Eruptions - comedones, chin
Eruptions - comedones, nose
Eruptions - herpes, circinatus
Eruptions - herpes, lips, about
Eruptions - pustules
Eruptions - pustules, chin
Eruptions - pustules, nose
Eruptions - pustules, nose, inside
Eruptions - spots
Expression - sickly
Greasy
Heat
Heat - chill, during
*Itching, lips*Swelling - lips
Swelling - lips, upper

Mouth:

Cracked - tongue
Discolouration - tongue, red
Discolouration - tongue, red stripe down centre
Dryness - tongue
Mucous - excoriation
Odour, offensive
Odour - putrid
Pain - sore, tongue
Speech - thick

Taste - metallic

Teeth:

Grinding - sleep, during

External throat:

Air - sensitive to
Goitre
Induration - like knotted cords
Induration - of glands
Swelling - cervical glands
Swelling - suppurative

Stomach:

Anxiety - capricious (doesn't know what to eat)
Appetite - ravenous, emaciation, with
Appetite, wanting, morning*Appetite - wanting, hunger, with*
Averse - food
Averse - food, hunger, with
Averse - meat
Desires - bacon
Desires - cold milk
Desires - delicacies
Desires - fat ham
Desires - ice cream
Desires - meat
Desires - meat, smoked
Desires - pork
Desires - refreshing things
Desires - salty things
Desires - sweets
Emptiness
Nausea - morning
Nausea - breakfast, before
Nausea, pressure, abdomen, on

Thirst - chill, during
Thirst - heat, during
Thirst - heat, after
Vomiting
Vomiting - bile
Vomiting - frothy
Vomiting - heat during
Vomiting - mucus
Vomiting - sour
Vomiting - sweetish

Abdomen:

Coldness
Enlarged - liver
Pain, pressing, hypogastrium, paroxysmal
Swelling - inguinal region, glands
Tabes mesenterica

Rectum:

Constipation
Constipation, alternating with diarrhoea
Constipation - painful
Diarrhoea - forenoon
Diarrhoea - morning
Diarrhoea - morning, driving out of bed
Diarrhoea - menses, after
Diarrhoea - menses, before
Diarrhoea - menses, during
Diarrhoea - motion agg
Diarrhoea - painless
Diarrhoea - sleep, during
Diarrhoea - weakness, without
Excoriation
Excoriation - stools, from the
Haemorrhage - stool, during
Haemorrhage - stool, from hard

Haemorrhoids
Haemorrhoids - chronic
Haemorrhoids, external
Haemorrhoids - large
Involuntary stool - flatus, passing
Involuntary stool - sleep, during
Itching
Pain - stool, during

Stool:

Acrid - corrosive, excoriating
Hard
Large
Lienteric
Light - coloured
Odour - offensive
Odour - putrid

Bladder:

Pain,desire be postponed, if
Retention - of urine
Urination, involuntary, night (incontinence in bed)

Urine:

Albuminous
Colour - red
Odour - ammoniacal
Odour - strong
Scanty
Sediment - sand

Genitalia - male:

Erection - child, in a
Masturbation - disposition

Relaxed - scrotum
Seminal emission, nightly
Sexual passion - excessive
Sexual passion - increased
Sexual passion - violent
Tubercles - testes

Genitalia - female:

Leucorrhoea - walking <
Masturbation - disposition
Menses - absent (amenorrhoea)
Menses - clotted
Menses - copious (menorrhagia)
Menses - delayed in girls, first menses
Menses - frequent (too early, too soon)
Menses - green
Menses - irregular
Menses - late
Menses - membranous
Menses - membranous, mental excitement <
Menses - painful (dysmenorrhoea)
Menses - protracted
Menses - thin
Metrorrhagia
Pain - cramping, uterus, menses, during
Pain - uterus, menses, during
Prolapse - uterus
Relaxation - of sphincter vaginae
Tumour - uterus, fibroids

Larynx:

Pain - rawness, larynx, cold air
Phthisis - larynx

Respiration:

Accelerated
Difficult
Difficult - night, during
Difficult - air, in open >
Difficult - exertion, after
Difficult - heat, with
Difficult - lying on back, impossible
Difficult - lying, while
Difficult - warm room, in a
Rattling

Cough:

Chill - before
Chill - during
Cold - drinks <
Cold - on becoming
Dry
Dry - sudden loss of breath, before chill
Fever - during
Hacking
Lying - side right
Reading - aloud <
Sleep - during
Suffocative
Talking
Talking - loud
Warm - room

Expectoration:

Greenish
Thick
Yellow

Chest:

Abscess - lungs
Cancer - mammae
Catarrh
Catarrh - old people
Hepatization - of lungs
Induration - mammae
Milk - disappearing
Milk, menses, before
Milk, menses, during
Milk, menses, suppressed
Milk, non-pregnant women
Milk - thin
Milk - thin and watery
Murmurs
Oppression
Pain
Pain - lungs
Pain - pinching
Pain - sore mammae, menses, before
Palpitation, heart,lying, side
Perspiration - axilla
Phthisis - incipient
Phthisis - pulmonalis
Swelling, mammae, menses, before
Swelling, mammae, menses, during
Swelling, mammae, secretion of milk, with
Ulcer - lungs

Back:

Stiffness
Stiffness - chill, during

Extremities:

Coldness - leg

Coldness - leg, evening, in bed
Coldness - leg, left
Coldness - leg, uncovering >
Hip - joint disease
Inflammation - knee
Ingrowing - toe nails
Lameness - foot
Pain - aching
Pain - aching, bones
Pain - aching, leg
Pain - aching, lower limbs
Pain - aching, thigh
Pain - burning, wrist
Pain - chill, during
Pain - coition, after
Pain - cold, weather
Pain - drawing, lower limbs
Pain - drawing, leg
Pain - fever, during
Pain - lower limbs, cold, becoming
Pain - lower limbs, motion >
Pain - lower limbs, paroxysmal
Pain - lower limbs, walking
Pain - leg
Pain - leg, chill, during
Pain - leg, cold, becoming
Pain - leg, motion >
Pain - leg, rheumatic, walking >
Pain - leg, warmth of bed >
Pain - motion >
Pain - sore, bruised
Pain - sore, bruised, joints
Pain - stitching, leg
Pain - stitching, lower limbs
Pain - tearing
Pain - tearing, joints
Pain - tearing, lower limbs
Pain - wandering, shifting

Pain - wet weather
Perspiration - hand, palm
Restless - leg
Spotted - nails
Stiffness - exertion, after
Swelling - knee
Trembling - hand
Twitching - one arm, one leg

Sleep:

Sleepiness
Sleeplessness - active mind

Chill:

Evening, in bed
Night
Noon
Annual - chill
Chilliness - perspiration, with
Creeping
Day - twenty eighth
5pm
7pm

Fever:

Night
Night, chilliness, after
Night, dry burning heat
Burning - heat
Chilliness - putting hands out of bed, from
Chilliness - with
Hectic - fever
Intense - heat
Intermittent - chronic
Perspiration - absent

Perspiration - heat with
Relapsing
Remittent - prone to become typhoid
Shivering - uncovering, from
Side - right
Succession - heat, followed by chill
Uncovering - aversion to
Uncovering - chilliness from

Perspiration:

Midnight, after
Clammy
Cold
Exertion - mental
Motion - brings on chilliness
Odour - foetid
Profuse
Single parts
Sleep - during
Stain - yellow
Uncovering - aversion
Writing - while

Skin:

Discolouration - brown, liver spots
Discolouration - dirty
Discolouration - yellow, intermittent fever, after
Eruptions
Eruptions - herpetic, circinate
Eruptions - itching, heat of stove >
Eruptions - leprosy
Eruptions - suppressed
Itching - heat of stove >
Itching - undressing <
Odour - foetid

Generalities:

Abscessess - glands

Change - of weather <

Change - weather, cold to warm <

Cold - place, entering <

Cold - tendency to take

Cold - wet weather <

Emaciation

Emaciation - pining boys

Exertion - physical <

Heat - flushes

Heat - flushes, perspiration with

Heat - vital lack of

Lean people

Pain - sore, bruised, on motion >

Pain - wandering

Periodicity - seventh day

Periodicity - twenty eighth day

Periodicity - twenty first day

Reaction - lack of

Sensitiveness - to pain

Standing - <

Stoop - shouldered

Storm - approach of a

Swelling - glands, knotted cords, like

Walking - <

Walking - fast >

Warm - bed >

Warm - room <

Weakness - (enervation)

Weakness - menses, during

Weakness - perspiration, from

Weariness

Wet - weather <

- 11 -
Tubercular Types

When we take the case an important section of the symptoms we must elicit are those which describe the disease traits or tendencies in the patient and his/her family. Very seldom do we come across uncomplicated cases and it is therefore important to be aware of those symptoms which indicate the mixture of miasms and therefore the nosodes likely to be needed. In patients such as these the stresses encountered in daily living, be they emotional or environmental, can be sufficient to precipitate a tubercular state.

1) Subject to continual colds and coughs - flu's. Intermittent fever. Febrile states without reason. Sore throats. Adenoids enlarged. Broncho-pneumonia. Coughs, < open air (Rumex).

2) Fatigue - weariness, > warm bed. Poor resistance. < Standing.(Sulphur). Work exhausts. Emaciation. Exhausted with respiratory troubles - too weak to speak (Stann).

3) Circumscribed cheeks - heat of face. Look younger than they are. Flushings and burnings of heat. Peripheral congestions. Long lashes with rosy complexion.

4) Irritability on waking. If children, even very little, are scolded they threaten back. Grumpy. Solitary. Critical and selfish. Peevish when ill. Angers followed by weakness. Negative.

5) Profuse perspiration at night or on exertion. Only perspires on the nose (peculiar and characteristic - Schmidt). Palms of hands damp.

6) Wants to travel constantly. Changing occupations. Hyperactive. > Open air and wind in face. < In cold weather. > In mountains. > Frosty, crisp air. Intense restlessness of mind and body. Rushes around to relieve tension.

7)   Symptoms constantly changing (Puls). Alternating states. Obstinate - contrary. Reckless - remorseful. > Before an aggravation - well the day before (Psor).

8)   Fear of dogs. Fear of cats. Fear of furry animals. Apprehensions.

9)   Desires smoked meats, sweets (Sulph), bacon, milk, wine, ice cream.

10) Sexual excitement excessive in very young boys. Violent.

11) Very sensitive mentally and physically. Imaginative. Creative. Love idealistic - beauty - harmony. Vulnerability. Weeps from music. Hypersensitive to pain. Hysterias. Susceptibility high to Rhus poisoning.

12) Chronic headaches. Menstrual headaches of intensity (Tub, Psor). Abnormal hunger before headaches (Phos, Psor). Periodicity - weekly, fortnightly. < Motion., from over-work, excitement, over-eating, before storm.

13) Skin eruptions > heat of stove. Acne. Pale pink scurf patches on skin and face.

14) Constipation. Tendency to liver upsets. Bleeding haemor-rhoids. Fistula of the anus (Psor). Large hard stools, then diarrhoea and sweating.

15) Chronic cystitis. Bright's disease. Nocturnal enuresis (1/3 of cases are Tub). Menses - too early - profuse, long lasting. Amenorrhoea. Dysmenorrhoea. Uterus sags - heavy. Pain in left testicle.

16) Acute articular rheumatism (Schlegel). Sore, bruised, aching all over the body - wandering. < Touch. Stiffness on begin-ning to move.

17) Teething in babes (Bell, Calc). Glands. Meningeal troubles (Tub). Frequent dental cases.

18) Wens of wrist and excessive synovial fluid of the knee (Calc, Tub). Ingrowing toe nails.(Psorinum). Callouses on soles of feet.(Psorinum).

19) Croup. Asthma. Hayfever. Ringworm. Goitre. Hacking coughs. Chill. Fever. Expectoration yellow/green. < Cold. Suffocation in a warm room. > In cold wind.

- 12 -
Tuberculinum Bovinum

Kent obtained it from a vet where cattle had been slaughtered for TB. It was potentised by Boericke and Skinner in the higher potencies. It should be used as any other remedy, ie on the indications of the sick person's symptom complex similar to the drug's pathogenesis.

1)   It is used, if according to indications, our well chosen remedy acts for only a few weeks.

2)   Prominent use in intermittent fevers. Stubborn cases of fever which continue to relapse. Causation from colds, sitting in a draft, becoming fatigued, mental exertion, over-eating. When a person has incipient TB. He has a febrile constitution and so complaints tend continually to relapse and remedies do not hold for long because of a deep seated tendency.

3)   Always tired. Debilitated. Emaciated. Weakness P.M. Become anaemic. Languid. Won't talk. Nervous - lassitude in stormy weather. All gone hungry feeling that drives one to eat (Sulph).

4)   Adenoids. Tuberculous glands of the neck. Axilla. Glands mesenteric. Inguinal.

5)   Hopelessness in many complaints. Weary of life. Aversion to mental work. Sulky. Complaining. Anxieties - evening, night, during fever. Loquacity during fever. Childrens' temper tantrums. Sensitivity to music. Changes quickly from one subject to another (Kent p63 add). Desires constant change, travel, to find somewhere else. Cosmopolitan (Calc-p). Persons on borderland of insanity (TB and insanity are convertible conditions). Lungs and intellect changeable.

Symptoms constantly changing about, needing different remedies.

6) Chronic sick headaches - weekly, fortnightly. Periodical nervous headaches. < Motion. Headaches from over-work (Calc-p). From mental excitement. From over-eating. (If headaches helped often the patient may get a persistent cough). Pain as of a tight band or hoop around head. Tubercular meningitis. Wakes frightened and screaming (Apis, Hell).

7) Sore bruised feeling all over body. Aching. < Damp. < Rest. Wandering aching of bones, periostium, legs. < Motion. Thighs. Soreness of eyeballs. Sensitive to touch > walking. Cold sweats on head. Aching bones of head. Stiffness on beginning to move (Rhus). Standing is much << (Sulph).

8) Constipation. Large hard stools then diarrhoea and sweating. Itching anus. Stitches in side after running.

9) Menses - too early, too profuse, longlasting. Amenorrhoea. Dysmenorrhoea. Uterus sags down and is heavy, as if would come out. Menses returns 14 days after childbirth. Pain, testicles, left side.

10) Hacking cough and chill and fever. Intermittent fever. Remedies cure but slightest exposure to cold and it returns. Suffocation in a warm room. > In cold wind. Desires to breathe deeply, > in cold air. Sits in room covered in sweat, > in cold air. (Then takes a cold). Expectoration yellow, yellow/green in catarrhal conditions.

11) Ringworm (Bacillinum). Formication. Red purplish eruptions nodular. Itching > near fire. Itching < cold air.

12) Jerking muscles on going to sleep and during sleep.

13) Desires milk, delicacies, smoked meat (Caust, Calc-p), bacon, pork, alcohol, ice cream.

14) < Every change in weather. < Before a storm, atmospheres. Periodicity. < Close room. > Cool open air (except skin). Aversion food, meat.

- 13 -
Collected Tips on the Treatment of the Tubercular Constitution

Nash   In advanced TB use Bacillinum or Tuberculinum high and let it act a long time without repetition.

Burnett   Bacillinum 100 - 200 can be used in acute fevers, frequently prescribed even up to once every two weeks. In early stages of tubercular disease of glands, joints, skin, bones. In advanced chronic cases preferably give Psorinum (Psorinum is the complementary of Bacillinum - Creasy.) Ars-i 3x-30c invaluable bd or tds.

Long   Tuberculinum Koch preferred in TB of the skin. Bacillinum selected for preference in consumptives had good results.

Kent   Choose Tuberculinum only if symptoms agree not just because it is TB. Feverish chills with cough where only smaller remedies help. Must have air.

Boericke   Advises Arsenicum iodatum to be given for some time in TB, beginning about 4x and gradually going lower to the 2x tds, 5 grains three times a day.

Boericke's recommendation of going lower in potency in successive prescriptions can be understood in terms of finding the potency which is appropriate to the patient. For ***similimum is remedy plus potency***. In my own practice if I have had disappointing results from 9c for example, I have often gone to a 3c and achieved far better results.

The Arsenicum iodatum picture is of corrosive discharge, profound prostration, rapid pulse, recurring fevers, diarrhoeas, night sweats, chilly, > air, emaciation, burnings, thick membrane in the throat from fauces to lips, discharges purulent - yellow or yellow/green, < A.M., < exertion, < ascending, < warm air, < warm bed, hurried, agitated, restless, loquacious, oversensitiveness and tormented, persistent thoughts.

Tendency to bleeding in TB (see Kent p814 - expectoration, bloody, streaked).
        Calc ars 3x, Ferr acet 1x, Nux-v, Mill.

Cough - spasmodic, retching, vomiting	Drosera 6, every 2 hours.
Frothy blood with nausea	Ipecac.
Frothy blood without cough	Millef 1x-30c every 15 mins - half hour.
Hectic fever	Ars iod.
Hoarse cough, rattling mucus, profuse yellow expectoration	Hepar 6.
Night sweats, constipation, loaded urine - odorous	Lycopodium.
Profuse perspiration, abundant sputa - sweet taste. WEAK.	Stann 6 - 30 - 1M.
Profuse perspiration	Jaborandi.
Rusty sputum	Phosphorus.

- 14 -
If Aggravation Follows the Giving of Tuberculinum in High Potency

Where the patient's disease has resulted in pathological changes, such that Tuberculinum high disturbs the system too much, these remedies will be of help. The remedy in this high potency which has provoked this over reaction may have been the indicated remedy but the patient's vitality, combined with the severity of the pathological changes, has not the capacity to throw off its own disease picture.

Bleeding from lungs (Haemoptysis)
Ferr-p 3x, Ferr-ac 1x, Mill. Repeating remedy and raising potency according to urgency.

Bleeding assoc. with fears
Aconite 30-1M, repeat according to urgency.

Bleeding of small amounts
Phos 30.

Cavities in lungs following chronic pneumonia
Bac 200, Ars-i 3-30 tds.

Chest pains
Myrtus communis.

Chronic inflammation of lungs (large parts), night sweats, loaded urine, constipation
Lycopodium 6.

Chronic (small) patches on lungs with rusty expectoration
Phos 30-200.

Consolidation of lung, rattling mucus, hoarse cough < night, profuse yellow expectoration	Hep 6-30, every 2 hours.
Expectoration of little granules	Kali-c 30-200.
Frothy blood without much cough (felt behind sternum). High temperature.	Mill 1x-200, hourly.

- 15 -
Tubercular Remedy Images

Spongia   Tubercular diathesis. High rasping cough.Croup. Wakes suddenly with anxious dyspnoea.Hard, chronically enlarged glands. Tubercular laryngitis (Dros). Severe forms of asthma.

Calc phos   Tall, scrawny children. Constant desire to be on the move. Restless. Peevish. Craves bacon rind. Slow dentition. Tearing pains in ears in cold. Child wants to nurse all the time.

Nat mur   Late walking and talking. Irritability. Delayed menses. Losing weight although eating well. Nervous weakness. Hypochondriacal anxiety. Anaemia. > Open air. < Heat. Malarial cachexia. Mucus hawking. Headaches. Weakness.

Stannum   Sad, despondent. Cries frequently. Faint. Short breath. Profuse sweats. Weakness. < Emotions. Sweet expectoration. Green. Coughs. Neuralgias. Menses profuse and early.

Agaricus   Late walking and talking. Rages. Twitching eyelids. Changeable. Nervous restlessness. Loquacious. > Nights, brighten up. < Morning. Stubborn. Headaches. Ecstatic. < Cold air. Ataxia. Growing pains.Prolapse, bearing down of uterus.

Iodum   Ravenous hunger yet emaciates. < Heat. > Air. Violent, wants to kill. Croupy coughs. Adenoids. TB.

Drosera

Aphonia. Tickling cough. Larynx hoarse. Barking. Sinusitis < 12A.M as head touches pillow. Growing pains. Epilepsy. Goitre. Anxieties. Irritable. > Company. > Open air. > Walking. Restlessness. Rheumatoid arthritis. Pain in long bones. Joints stiff. Hip sore. History of TB going to insanity.

Nat ars

Aches all over, > quiet. Night sweats. Fevers. Restless. Chilly. Nervous. Catarrhs. Nose blocked A.M. - mouth breather. Dark red, swollen, purple throat. Suppuration. Copious green expectoration. Chest as if full of smoke. Compressive pain at root of nose.

- 16 -
Tubercular Remedies

From EA Farrington's Clinical Materia Medica:

Lachesis is useful in the latter stages of pneumonia especially when an abscess forms on the lungs. Muttering, delirium and hallucinations appear. The sputum is frothy, mixed with blood, purulent and the patient is bathed in sweat.

It can be used in tuberculosis, not necessarily to cure but to relieve, even in advanced stages when the person retches with the cough which rouses him from sleep ending with tough, greenish, muco-purulent matter, which causes gagging, and is vomited rather than clearly expectorated; when the patient sweats during every nap. Extreme prostration.

Sulphur is perhaps the better remedy to prevent suppuration when there are no typhoid symptoms as above. But be careful how you give Sulphur if tuberculosis has been developed by pneumonia. To do so is almost like giving a person running downhill another push. It will only hasten the end.

Iodoformum is very useful for TB conditions especially tubercular meningitis and for failing eyesight (retro bulbar neuritis)- atrophy of optic disc. Loss of strength - malaise. Pupils contracted unequally. Mesenteric glands enlarged. Loss of appetite. Chronic diarrhoea - stools greenish, watery and undigested. Drowsiness constant (Op). < Night, warmth. Exalted ideas. Loquacity. Excitement - melancholia - hallucinations of sight and hearing. Screams out. Talks nonsense. Delusions.

Iodum: glands - thyroid, testes, mesenteric, mammary.
1) Swollen, hard, heavy.
2) Dwindle.

Always feels too hot.
Weak - looses flesh. Debilitated. Any effort induces perspiration.
Cannot talk. Out of breath going up stairs.
Oedema - vasoconstriction - haemmorhages.
Adenoids. TB. Tickly, croupy cough.
General pulsations or throbbings in arteries.
Burnings.
Restless. Dejected. Weepiness. Irritable. Anxieties.
Wants to do violence. Wants to kill.
< Motion.
Fears people.
Suicidal.
Ravenous hunger yet emaciates.

Blatta orientalis (Indian cockroach):
Useful in cases of bronchitis and TB where there is much dyspnoea.
Relieves asthma (low potencies).
< Rainy weather.
Suffocation threatened by accumulation of mucus.

Blatta Americana (American cockroach):
Acute pain in chest with want of breath. General prostration going upstairs.
Jaundice.

Agaricus:
Numerous and diverse symptoms.
Tremblings, twitchings, nervousness, restlessness.
Chorea.
Sensation of ice cold needles.
Excitable.
Loquacious - makes verses and rhymes. Ecstatic.
Awkward, clumsy.
Does opposite to routine work.
Stubborn.
Brain complaints.
Children walk too late.
Headache - moves head to and fro (Tub).

Epilepsy. Chillblains and bunions.

Natrum arsenicum:
Hectic fever, night sweats, coughing, copious green expectoration, purulent expectoration.
It is like Arsenicum in that it is restless and chilly.
They are depressed, lustreless, nervous, restless.

Catarrhs	-	nose stuffed up in morning - mouth breather (Ant-t, Lach, Lyc, Op, Samb, Sulph).
	-	post nasal drip, yellow mucus.
	-	hawking, greeny-yellow expectoration.
Throat	-	dark red and swollen, covered with yellow mucus.
	-	purple throat, swelling, little pain.
Bronchitis	-	oppressive chest, as if full of smoke.
Nose	-	compressive pain at root.
	-	aching over brows, orbits and temples < waking.
Eyes	-	conjunctivitis.
	-	smarting, inflammed.
Generals	-	tired, achy all over.
	-	wants to be quiet.
	-	< On moving.
	-	< During day.
	-	> Quiet.
	-	Chilliness.
	-	Thirst.

- 17 -
Tubercular - Sycotic

Remedies related to Selenium and their associated miasmatic influences

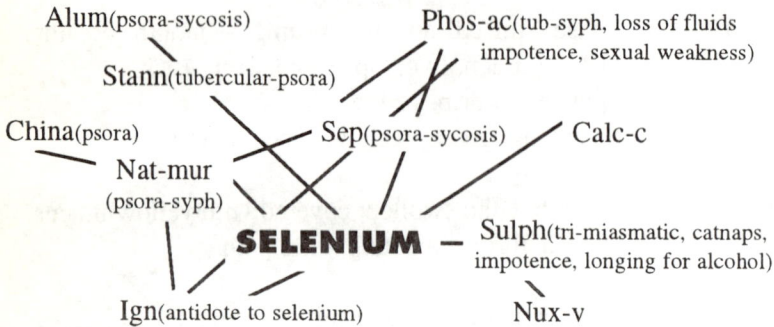

Alum(psora-sycosis)

Phos-ac(tub-syph, loss of fluids impotence, sexual weakness)

Stann(tubercular-psora)

China(psora)

Sep(psora-sycosis)

Calc-c

Nat-mur
(psora-syph)

SELENIUM — Sulph(tri-miasmatic, catnaps, impotence, longing for alcohol)

Ign(antidote to selenium)

Nux-v

Selenium:

Cannot take any nervous drain - weakness from prolonged fever.
Asthenic remedy. From anger.
Weakness of memory.
Loss of hair - eyebrows, hair, whiskers.
Juvenile acne - psoriasis between fingers, palms.
Weakness. Suddenly overcome, > lying down.
< Hot weather or from fluid loss.
Constipation. Impacted faeces (Sanic, Op).
Mucus in throat. Hoarseness. Tubercular laryngitis.
Frequent clearance of throat, of starchy mucus (Spong, Caust, Carbo-v, Phos).
Female - copious, dark menses. Irritable after coition.
Male - impotence with strong sexual desire (Con, Phos). Sexual emissions frequent. Secondary gonorrhoea. Craves stimulants. Erections insufficient. Irritable after coition.
Headache - nervous, left eye, < tea, sharp stitches left eye.
Generals   - < Drafts, strong odours, tea, coffee.
            - < Hot days, sun, wine, fluid loss (sweats, sex, mastur-
              bation) illness.
            - > After sunset, cool, lying down

Tubercular - Syphilitic

Remedies related to Hippozaeninum.

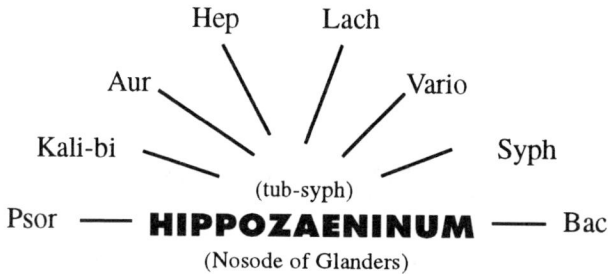

```
              Hep        Lach
      Aur        \        /        Vario
  Kali-bi  \      \      /      /
             \     \    /    /        Syph
              \     \  /  /  /
               (tub-syph)
  Psor ——  HIPPOZAENINUM  —— Bac
         (Nosode of Glanders)
```

Hippozaeninum:

Suppurations - catarrhs, inveterate and of the glands. Bronchitis. Hoarseness, frontal sinus, pharynx, larynx, trachea, bronchial asthma. Whooping cough. Long-term coughs (Sang).

Glands. Ulcerations (mouth, nose, tonsils, abdomen, hepatitis, gall ducts). Abscesses.
TB diminishes expectoration, abates constantly, recurring aggravations of inflammation. Lung disease of cattle.
Elephantiasis.
Weakness.

Tubercular - Psoric

Remedies related to Calcarea iodatum

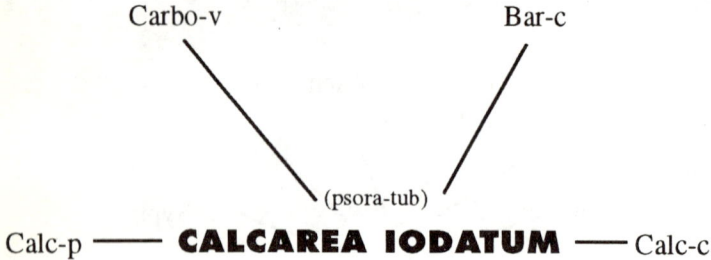

Carbo-v   Bar-c

(psora-tub)

Calc-p —— **CALCAREA IODATUM** —— Calc-c

Calcarea iodatum:
Rather like Calc-c in characteristics but scraggy, with enormous appetite.
> Meals (not Calc-c).
> Open air.
< Hot rooms.
Gets angered easily.
Anxious worriers.
Indifference.
Indolence.
Glandular enlargements.
Nodules in breast, breast tumours - movable, < touch (tender).
Enlarged tonsils.
TB of glands.

Catarrhal Tuberculosis

Silica   In catarrhal and pulmonary TB. Copious rattling phlegm. Purulent expectoration (more so than Stann). Especially indicated in catarrhal TB of the elderly.

Stannum   From neglected colds. Must have weakness or it will fail. Feverishness (hectic). Chills 10am. Hot and flushed in evenings. Sweats at night. Sweet or greenish expectoration.

Coccus cacti Catarrhal TB. Ropy phlegm. Sharp, stitching pains under clavicles.

Formica rufa TB. Cancer. Gout. Rheumatics.

Selenium   Tubercular laryngitis. Asthenic remedy. < Sun.

Bloody mucus - it is still possible to cure if there is not complete destruction of lungs.

First stages of tubercular, pulmonary:
Calc, Phos, Hep, Spong. (Jahr).

Pulmonary haemorrhage:
Ip, Chin, Ferr, Bry, Acon, Arn, Ars.

Tuberculosis:
Acon, Arn, Phos, Ph-ac (in late stage), Sep, Mill.

Hawking blood:
Acon, Ip, Nux-v, Sulph, Ars.

Racking cough:
Chin, Ip, Nux-v.

If (blood) vomited without a cough:
Ip, Arn, Phos, Chin, Ars, Ferr.

< Night:
Ferr, Puls, Rhus-t, Sel, Hyos.

< During rest:
Rhus, Dulc.

< After exercise:
Bry, Ferr, Bell, Chin.

< After talking:
Phos, Ferr.

< In morning especially:
Phos, Ars, Chin, Nux-v.

If blood bright red:
Dulc, Rhus-t, Acon, Arn, Bell, Ferr, Ip, Chin, Ars.

If blood dark, blackish:
Arn, Puls, Sec.

If blood slimy, thick and viscid:
Arn, Op, Rhus-t.

Hoarseness:
Phos, Chin, Sulph.

Burning in the chest:
Carb-v, Arn, Ars.

Weakness:
Arn, Ars.

Incipient TB with pains between the shoulder blades or in the region of the clavicle. Frequent dry cough. Setting in especially in the evening, at bed time or early hours of the morning with few blood streaks in the sputa,:
Bry, Calc-c, Lyc, Nux-v, Phos, Sulph, Chin, Ip, Hep, Spong, Dros.

Briny mucus:
Spong, Bac.

Frothy blood with nausea and tickling cough:
Ipecac 6-30 hourly

Weakness expectoration of abundant yellow/green sputa, sweetish taste:
Stannum 30-200.

- 21 -
Pulmonary Tuberculosis Cases Remedy Reactions

1) Cough, temperature, night sweats and haemoptysis have increased with further loss of weight and no appetite. This is deteriorating, and a quick change of remedy or remedies are needed.

2) If after giving the homœopathic remedy the aggravation persists for a long time. This will deteriorate within the progression of the disease yet further.

3) A gradual decline without improvement is not a good sign after a remedy for it means that the vital force is not capable of reaction, after being stimulated, the pathology is dominant. The possibilities of cure will need persistent use of LM potencies, so that the vital force may be gently aroused to a level of strength.

4) High potencies - in these cases I do not recommend them. Rather gradually increase the potency by Hahnemann's plussing method in water, or change to the LM's. This way of giving remedies is far kinder in deep pathological cases.

5) If a constitutional remedy is given there will be a lot of undulating improvements and declines in the case. Intercurrent remedies usually revolving around the constitution are frequently required.
Intercurrents frequently take the edge off remedies if acting too deeply (acute relationships) ie. alleviate excessive reaction of the vital force to the deep acting remedy without hindering the deep acting remedy's curative process due to their complementary nature.

6)   The shifting of remedies in certain chronic cases is justifiable. Hahnemann, Kent and Burnett all did this. In a mixture of the miasms, where one miasm is improved for a while under a deep remedy. For instance the psoric may be improved first at which point the second miasm starts emerging, requiring a different chronic remedy. Some cases require a succession of remedies until the economy is balanced, until one remedy is finally found.

7)   In cases of utter weakness, Stannum and Phosphoric acid are especially to be mentioned and Phosphoric acid to be used instead of Phosphorus in these cases.

8)   Any old symptom that recurs and persists needs to be high on the evaluation for the next choice of remedy.

9)   Cases with irreversible organ changes may need palliation only. However many of these cases if nurtured along come back to curability.

10)   Suppress any form of ringworm and there often follows tubercular disease. (Burnett).

Epilepsy - psoric or tubercular diathesis.
Dysmenorrhoea - mania, PMT - tubercular.

Tubercular latent	Hair dry and lustreless
(observations)	Dental arch imperfect
	Teeth malformed
	Pale face flushes easily
Syphilitic side	Eyelashes stubby and broken
	Lids of eyes scaly and red
	Hands and feet cold and clammy
	Nails thin and imperfect, split easily

11)   Morning diarrhoea in consumptives - Tub.

12)   Wakens with greenish expectoration - Kali-i, Merc-i-r, Puls, Psor, Stann.

13) Dyspnoea   < Wheezing and nausea   Ip

               < Lying down   Act-spic, Aral, Ars, Grind, Lach, Merc, Sulph, Puls, Sep, Stryc.

               < Lying left side   Naja, Spig, Tab, Visc.

               < Lying right side   Visc.

               < Rest   Sil.

               < Sitting up   Carbo-v, Laur, Psor, Sep.

- 22 -
Remedies Indicated
in Early Stages of TB

Phos - hereditary tendency
Oleum jecoris*
Ferr-met
Carb-an
Iod
Kali-c (right lobe affected)
Caust
Coc-c
Rumex
Sang
Spong
Codeinum
Stann
Sulph
Bac (Burnett)
Ars-iod*
Nat-ars*
Elaps
Hep

Borax
Brom
Ipecac* (haemoptysis)
Kali-i
Calc-p
Puls
Phos
Phos-ac
Sep (all three lobes affected)
Sil (suppurative stage)
Con
Dros
Laur
Manganum
Myritis
Nat-s
Ferr-p
Senega

* Remedies which are particularly useful

- 23 -
Remedies Indicated
in Later Stages of TB

Ars - last stages
Calc-c
Nit-ac
Guiacum - last stages
Psor (Burnett)

Bapt
Lach
Carb-an (bronchitis, late stage)
Pix liquida (3rd stage).

Warnings

Do not give Ars in early stages as the disease progresses down into the lungs.

Do not repeat Kali-c too often and not when the tubercles are formed.

Sulphur can be given high at the onset but in later stages after tubercles have formed do not repeat frequently. You must be certain of the remedy.

- 24 -
Tuberculinum - a Comparison

- Margaret Burgess-Webster MD.
- Hom.Rec. 1933 2nd Feb

Appetite good - enjoys food but loses weight:
Tub, Abrot, Iod, Nat-m, Ars-i.

Nervous, faint, must eat at once, so hungry gets up at night to eat:
Tub, Chin, Lyc, Phos, Psor.

Desires smoked beef, salted meats:
Tub, Caust, Kreos.

Desires stimulants, sweets, refreshing things:
Tub, Phos-ac, Sabad.

Desires cold milk:
Tub, Chel, Phos, Phos-ac, Rhus-t, Sanic.

Desires highly seasoned foods - salty and acids:
Tub, Med, Syph.

Desires warm foods and fats:
Tub, Nit-ac, Nux, Mez, Rad-brom.

Aversion to meat - impossible to eat:
Tub, Sanic, Sulph, Syph.

Aversion to smell of coffee:
Tub, Lach.

Nodes in breast:
Tub, Con, Iod, Phyt, Sil, Carb-an.

Annual and monthly attacks of flu:
    Tub.

Takes cold easily:
    Bac, Ars-i, Calc-p, Kali-c, Psor, Tub.

Mucus rattling in chest without expectoration:
    Ant-t, Tub.

Purulent expectoration:
    Bac, Tub, Ars-i, Kali-c, Psor.

Lack of reaction after pneumonia:
    Tub, Carb-v, Chin, Phos, Psor.

Palpitation early A.M. - beats so hard can be felt all over body:
    Tub, Nat-m.

Fluttering, valvular insufficiency, < lying left side, < lying down, >
sitting up on 3 pillows, sensation of heaviness and pressure, aching,
< waking:
    Tub.

Mesenteric glands swollen:
    Tub, Ars-i, Bac.

Cervical glands swollen:
    Tub, Bac, Kali-c, Psor.

Ringworm of scalp:
    Bac, Tub.

Deep in brain headaches:
    Bac, Tub, Psor.

Schoolgirl headaches:
    Tub, Calc-p.

Cramping pains in stomach with pressure, vomiting with nausea, repugnance at sight or odour of food and cooking:
Tub, Colch.

Many bowel and stomach disturbances, rectal haemorrhage, gas and torpidity, constipation for years - painful:
Lac-d, Syph, Tub.

Fissures rectum:
Tub, Thuj, Syph.

Faecal impaction:
Tub.

Diarrhoea - gushing pop-gun discharge:
Tub, Sulph, Pod, Crot-t.

Early A.M. diarrhoea - drives them out of bed:
Bac, Tub, Ars, Sulph, Iod, Kali-c, Psor, Pod.

Early A.M. diarrhoea - green and spluttering:
Calc-p, Bac, Tub.

Grinds teeth in sleep:
Bac, Tub, Kali-c, Psor.

Sleepless, disturbed around 3 A.M.:
Tub, Thuj, Ars.

Uterus - heavy, sagged, prolapse, < standing, must move:
Tub, Sep, Sulph.

Menses - gushing, clotted, profuse, exhausting, faints, frightful dysmenorrhoea:
Calc-c, Tub, Med, Lach.

Offensive leucorrhoea - brown, profuse:
Alum, Onos, Syph, Tub.

Remedies Related to Tuberculinum and their use in the Treatment of Tubercular Conditions

Information collected from the works of Lippe, Kent, Farrington, Burnett, Nash and Pulford.

Agaricus	Incipient TB, anaemia, neuralgias.
Agraphis	Catarrhs, obstruction, adenoids, throat, deafness, ear troubles.
Allium sativa	Liver types, pulmonary TB, haemoptysis, mucus rattles, sharp pains in chest.
Alumen	Haemoptysis, induration of glands tending to ulceration, marble like mass stools, constipation with no desire, piles.
Ars iod	Early stages of TB. Even where there is afternoon rise in temperature it is very effective. Prostration, recurrences, diarrhoeas, chronic pneumonias with abscess on lung. Persistent corrosive discharges. Old catarrhs, hypertrophied conditions of eustachian tube and deafness. Night sweats, pulmonary TB. Chronic bronchitis. > Open air.
Balsamum	Bronchial catarrh, chronic foetid nasal catarrh. Peruvianum TB with muco purulent, thick and creamy expectoration - loud rales (Kali-s, Ant-t). Loose cough, hectic fever, night sweats. Irritating short cough.

Baryta carb	Related to Psorinum in lung conditions. Suffocative cough in elderly.
Baryta mur	Mouth breathers, stupid, hard of hearing bronchial, elderly. Needs repetition.
Beta vulg	Chronic catarrh and TB. Excellent for children.
Blatta orientalis	Asthma especially when associated with bronchitis. Cough with dyspnoea. TB. Pus like mucus. Low potency during asthma attack,higher later.
Boletus laricis	Night sweats in TB. Hectic chills and fever.
Calc carb	Anti-psoric history. Affinity for the glands, skin, bones. Incipient TB (Ars iod, Tub). Polypi. Persistent sour taste. Bleeding gums. Bloody expectoration - tight chest, dyspnoea > fresh air. Salty and sweet expectoration. Abscess in lungs. Night terrors (Kali-p).
Calc fluor	TB, croup, expectoration of tiny yellow lumps. Indurations, stony hardness. Exhausting night sweats. Cough of TB. Bleeding from lungs. Cold extremities. Related: China.
Calc iod	Chronic cough. Enlarged glands, tonsils. Hectic fever, green purulent expectoration.
Calc phos	TB. Anaemia. Glands. Hoarseness. Diarrhoea and cough. Night sweats. > Lying down. Related: China, Nat-m.
Calc sil	Very sensitive to cold. Chilly but < being overheated. Emaciated. Difficult respiration - irritation. Copious yellow/green mucus. Pain in the chest. Flow between menses. Depressions. Fearful.

Calotropis	TB of the syphilitic miasm if Mercury cannot be used any further. Feels heat in the stomach.
Carbo veg	Burning in the chest with haemoptysis. Destructive lung disease. Thick yellow expectoration. Neglected pneumonia. Hoarseness < evening. Related: Kali-c, Dros.
China	Haemorrhage from lungs. Laboured, slow respiration. Suffocative catarrh, dyspnoea, rattling in chest. Night sweats. Drowsy. Related: Ferr, Calc-p, Carb-v, Kali-c.
Drosera	Laryngeal TB. Pulmonary TB. TB glands. Profuse yellow expectoration. Epistaxis, bleeding from the mouth. Rapid emaciation. Hoarseness. Paroxysms of cough follow each other rapidly. > Open air, cold, rest, sitting up.
Eriodictyon	Bronchial TB. Night sweats, emaciation, wheezing, profuse sputum easily raised. (Whooping cough).
Ferr phos	Pulmonary TB, acute first stage, inflammatory, haemoptysis - blood streaked sputum. Short, painful tickling cough. Hard, dry cough - sore chest. Hoarseness. Recurrent attacks of acute bronchitis. Epistaxis. Pure blood in the chest (Mill). Nervous, sensitive, easy flushing. < Night, 4-6 A.M. > Cold applications.
Ficus religiosa	Haemoptysis. Difficult respiration. Vomits blood. Compare: Mill, Ipecac.
Formic acid	Muscular soreness and pains. TB. Chronic nephritis. Related: Bac, Psor.

Gallicum ac.	Haematuria. TB. Pulmonary haemorrhage. Excessive expectoration - much mucus in the throat A.M. Compare: Phos.
Graphites	Chronic hoarseness. Skin.
Hamamelis	Haemoptysis. Tickling cough. Chest sore and restricted. Complementary: Ferr.
Hippozaeninum	(Nosode of glanders, a disease of horses). TB. Cancer. Chronic rhinitis. Hoarseness. Cough with dyspepsia. Suffocative cough. Lymphatic swellings. Nodules under arms. Ulcers. Compare: Aur, Kali-bi, Psor, Bac.
Inula	Palliative in tubercular laryngitis.
Iodoformum	TB conditions. Acute and chronic diarrhoea of children with suspected TB. Weakness. Haemoptysis. Cough, wheezing, as of a weight on the chest. Pain in the left breast. Relieves asthmatic conditions. Acute meningitis.
Iodum	Emaciation with great appetite. > After eating. Great debility. Any effort causes perspiration. Enlarged lymphatic glands. Tubercular type. Must keep busy. Nasal engorgement. Blood streaked mucus. Tickling larynx. Colds descend. < Warm room, > walking about, open air. Related: Brom, Hep, Merc, Phos, Nat-m, Sanic, Tub.
Ipecac	Haemoptysis, < from slightest exertion. Chest full of phlegm. Bubbling rales. Suffocative cough. (Whooping cough with nose bleed). Best remedy for constriction of the chest, wheezing. > Open air.

Kali carb	TB diathesis. Irritable. Dislikes being alone. Obstinate. Hypersensitive. Nose stuffs up in a warm room. Hoarseness. Stitching pains in the chest, > leaning forward. Coughs up cheesy lumps. Offensive sputa. Wheezing. Recurrent colds. Related:Calc-c, Carbo-v, Phos, Stann, Sep, Lyc.
Kali nitricum	Debility and relapse in TB. Hoarseness. Expectorates clotted blood after hawking. > Sips.
Kali iod	Air hunger. Early diarrhoea of TB. Stubborn chronicity. Glands enlarged and indurated. Hard lumps like nodes on the scalp. Coryza leading to sinusitis. Stitching pains. Pulmonary TB with violent racking cough, < in the morning, with frothy expectoration. Night sweats. < Heat, night. > Open air, motion.
Lachnanthes	Early stages of TB and established chest cases. Loquacity. Circumscribed red cheeks. Chilliness between shoulder blades. Stiffness. Tendency to sweat. Neck drawn to one side in sore throat - as if dislocated. Septic throats. In TB the mother tincture can be administered once or twice a week in unit doses or in emergencies three drops every four hours.
Lactic acid	Tubercular ulceration of vocal chords as of a lump in the throat. Keeps swallowing.
Lycopodium	Tubercular laryngitis especially when ulceration starts. Tickling cough. Dyspnoea. Expectoration - thick, grey, bloody, purulent - salty (Ars, Phos, Puls). Night cough as from sulphur fumes. Constriction of chest, burning in chest. Stitches and dryness to throat, > warm drinks. Stuffed up nose, snuffles, fluent coryza, ulcerated nostrils,

crusts. Chills and sweats - offensive axillae and feet.

Manganum Tuberculosis of larynx (Calc-c, Carbo-v, Kali-bi, Phos, Sulph). Chronic hoarseness. Cough, < evening, > lying down. Great accumulation of mucus. Soreness, aching. Haemoptysis. Every cold arouses bronchitis. Nose dry, obstructed.

Medorrhinum Incipient TB. Sore larynx. Dyspnoea. Pain, soreness of chest and mammae. Chronic nasal and pharyngeal catarrhs . In fever wants to be fanned. Hectic night sweats. Craves liquor salts, sweets. Throat is sore and swollen, deglutition of liquids or solids is impossible (Merc). Throat constantly filled with thick, grey, bloody mucus, from posterior nares (Hydras). Sputum difficult to raise. Incessant dry cough at night. Related: Thuja, Sulph, Syph.

Myrtus com. Chest pains as often found in consumptives. Dry hollow cough. Tickling < A.M. Burning.

Naphthalin Pulmonary TB. Gonorrhoea. Whooping cough. Terrible, offensive, ammoniacal urine. Acute laryngo-tracheitis. Tenacious expectoration. Hayfever. Related: Dros.

Oleum santali Two drops of the tincture on sugar to relieve hacking cough - little sputum.

Oxalic acid TB. Violent pains in spots, < motion and thinking of the pains. Dyspnoea. Left lung painful. Burning sensation in throat extending downwards. Hoarseness.

Phosphorus TB. Do not use too low or repeat too frequently. Haemoptysis (Ferr-p, Ip, Lach, Nit-ac, Sul-ac).

Incipient and more advanced TB. Oppression of chest. Rusty sputum. Hoarseness. Left lung, < lying on left side. Pain in larynx. Tightness in chest, as of a weight. Heat in chest. Tickling cough, < cold air, talking. Sweetish taste. Tuberculinum follows well and is complementary. Related: Chin, Sep, Lyc, Sulph.

Pilocarpus jaborandi Profuse sweats at night of consumptives (Populus trem). Foamy sputa. Painless diarrhoea.

Psorinum Often gives immunity to catching colds. Debility. Easy perspiration when walking. Quinsy extending to ears. Hawking of mucus, disgusting taste. Complementary: Tub, Sulph, Sep.

Stannum TB. Hectic fever. Weakness. Copious green, sweet expectoration. Cough excited by laughing and talking. Chest weak and can hardly talk. Stitches to left side when breathing and lying on it. Exhausting night sweats especially towards morning, hectic, smells musty and offensive. > Expectoration. Complementary: Puls, Calc-c, Bac, Tub.

Zinc met Related to Tuberculinum.

Dunham and Lippe consider Calc-c, Merc, Nit-ac, Phos, Puls, Sep, Sil and Sulph are related to Tuberculinum.

- 26 -
Farrington Remedies to be Found Useful in TB and Allied Conditions

Although most of you will not have seen cases of "open TB" it is prevalent in many parts of the world and is increasing in incidence in our inner cities. For the present, however, what may be of more significance is the tubercular diathesis which lurks behind many conditions we see. The lists of remedies which Farrington gives for bronchial catarrh and for use in TB itself are not only important in these states but recurring indications for these remedies demonstrates the tubercular diathesis. When such patients are exposed to environmental conditions such as malnutrition, over crowding, repeated chills, etc. they will be predisposed to tuberculosis.

Bronchial catarrh - a frequent symptom of TB and the pre-tubercular state

Ant tart   Cyanotic symptoms. Dyspnoea. Child cannot feed. Cries with cough. Cough when angry.

Arsenicum   Dry cough, frothy sputum, emphysematous dyspnoea.

Baryta carb   Glands of neck enlarged. Enlarged lymph nodes to bronchi.

Calc carb   Rattling mucus, loose cough.

Conium   Dry teasing cough, < lying.

Hepar sulph   Croupy. Harsh even though loose.

Iodum   Croupy, hoarse, < warm weather.

Kali carb   Stitches. Shortness of breath. Pus globules in sputum.

Kali iod   Lungs hepatised. Green, frothy sputum, looks like soap suds.

Lycopodium   Loose rattling cough. Moist rales. Yellow purulent sputum (Sulph).

Oleum jecoris   Lungs hepatised. Green, frothy sputum, looks like soap suds.

Phosphorus   Violent cough, quick breathing. Oppression of the chest. Cough plus diarrhoea. Hoarseness.

Sepia   Dry cough causes bilious vomiting.

Silica   Pain under the sternum. Rachitic children. Loose cough. Purulent sputum. Night sweats.

Sulphur   Dry cough. Flushes of heat. Rattling mucus, purulent yellow sputum.

Sulphuric acid Belches when coughing.

Bloody sputum:
Arg-nit, Ars, Phos, Sep, Sil, Merc.

Bright red bloody expectoration:
Acon, Arn, Ars, Bell, Bry, Carbo-v, Chin, Dros, Dulc, Ferr, Ferr-p, Ferr-a, Hyos, Ip, Kali-bi, Laur, Merc, Mill, Nit-ac, Nux-v, Phos, Puls, Rhus-t, Sabad, Sabin, Sec, Sep, Sil, Zinc.

Dark red bloody expectoration:
Acon, Arn, Bell, Bry, Carbo-v, Cham, Chin, Croc, Dros, Elaps, Ferr, Ferr-p, Ferr-a, Lyc, Merc, Nit-ac, Nux-v, Phos, Phos-ac, Sec, Sep, Puls, Sulph, Sul-ac.

Other remedies recommended by Farrington in TB and pre-tubercular conditions

Borax   Cough plus sharp stitching pains - catches breath. Expectoration musty, mouldy odour and taste.

Bromine   Right lung. Congestion of head and chest. > Nose bleed. Pain in mammary region extending to axilla.

Calc phos   Like Calc carb.

Carbo animalis Generally affects right lung. < Closing eyes = smothering. Later stages of bronchitis. Expectoration green, offensive. Cold feeling in chest.

Causticum   Hoarseness, < A.M. (Carbo-v, Phos < evening). Laryngeal weakness. Cannot cough deeply enough to raise the sputum - slips back into pharynx (Arn, Dros, Kali-c, Sep). > Drinking cold water.

Coccus cacti Catarrhal TB. Sore, sharp pains to lungs. Ropy phlegm - long strings.

Codeinum   Cough - annoys, dry, teasing, day and night.

Conium   Impossible to expectorate, must swallow it again. Tormenting night cough, dry spot, > as soon as sitting up.

Drosera   Spasmodic TB cough, < evening and midnight - retches. (Useful in asthma).

Elaps   Right lung (but may be both) intense pain in the chest. Pain A.M. Sputum dark, black blood.

Ferr phos   Prostrated. Blood streaked expectoration. Will quickly quieten pulmonary congestion.

Hepar sulph	Follows Spongia when same cough continues with more rattling. Mucus blood streaked. < Towards A.M.
Iodum	Persons who grow rapidly like Phos. Congestion of lungs is frequent. Emaciated with good appetite. Dry cough, tickling all over the chest. Tough, blood streaked expectoration. Weakness of chest especially going down stairs.< Warm room.
Kali iod	Frothy expectoration, soap suds, greenish. Night sweats. Loose stools A.M. Cough - violent, rattling, tearing < 3-5 A.M.
Laurocerasus	Dry teasing cough, < night. Expectoration with specks of blood. Lack of reaction to remedies.
Manganum	TB of larynx (Arg-n). Hoarseness, < A.M., > hawking.
Mephites	Asthma of TB when Dros fails (Nat-s).
Myrtus com	Pain in upper part of left chest extending through to shoulder blade.
Nat ars	Of great service in emaciation of TB. Dry heat of the skin. Chilliness at night. Thirst for frequent sips.
Nat sulph	Lower lobe of left lung, pain between 9th and 10th ribs. Cough with muco-purulent expectoration.
Phos ac	Great weakness - cannot talk. Dyspnoea. < Drafts. Wraps up warmly.
Phosphorus	Hereditary tendencies to TB or bone diseases from childhood. Remedy indicated more in general character. Catches colds easily. Tight,constrictive feeling in chest, > sitting up. Pains in left lung. Hoarseness.

Dry cough. Haemoptysis. Hectic flush to cheeks, < evenings. Thirst for cold drinks. < 10-11 A.M. Hungry at night. Early childhood like Calc-c. Chronic tendency to diarrhoea.

Senega   Especially indicated in fat people (Calc-c). Soreness of chest, < moving arms, esp. left. Accumulation of mucus with difficult expectoration. Pressure on chest, feels pushed in. Blocked nose. > Bending back, < A.M, night, motion.

Sepia   Indicated when all three lobes of the lung are affected (Calc-c, Calc-p).

Silica   Catarrhal, copious rattly phlegm - suppurative stage (more purulent than Stann). Offensive. Cough at first dry becomes loose. Old people especially.

Stannum   Catarrhal - rarely true TB. Oppression of chest, tightness, > expectoration (easy), weakness. Teasing cough, tenacious mucus with a little blood accumulating in the throat. Hoarseness. Dyspnoea, > towards A.M. Fever, < 10 A.M. Flushed, hot. Profuse night sweats < 4-5 A.M. Depressed. Followed well by Coc-c, Phos, Seneg, Sil.

Remedies particularly indicated in the early/ incipient stages of TB

Ferr met   Appearence of blooming health of TB subjects in the incipient stages (Phos). Oppression of the chest, < any exertion. Nostrils dilate with the effort to breathe. Frequent epistaxis and haemoptysis - blood bright red, coagulated. Dry teasing cough after warm drinks plus sore, bruised feeling in chest and dull aching pain to occiput. Expectoration - greenish and odorous.

Ipecac

Best remedy in haemoptysis of incipient TB. Profuse bright blood plus nausea. Hard, laboured breathing. Cold sweats.

Kali carb

Face bloated, puffiness - upper eyelids. Stitching pains lower third of right lung extending from chest through to back. Expectoration difficult, bloody. < 3-5 A.M. Stubborn. Useful when TB threatens at puberty (Calc-c). Do not repeat too often and not when tubercles have formed.

Oleum jecoris

Chills up and down spine. Hoarseness, soreness of chest. Burning in spots and on palms of hands. Fever, < evening. Cough dry. Shiny mucus.

Pulsatilla

Especially indicated at puberty before the menses are established or where periods are retarded. Sore chest, burning around heart. Stitches. Cough with expectoration - bloody.

Rumex

Stitches, stinging pains in the chest, left lung. Left side sore, < turning.

Sanguinaria

The early stages of "galloping consumption". Hectic fever 2-4 P.M. Cheeks red, circumscribed. Cough dry, tickling in larynx, burning, fulness congestion. Stitches, especially right lung extending to nipple. Chest muscles sore. Dyspnoea. Laryngeal catarrh.

Spongia

TB of the lungs, especially the first stage of solidification of lung tissue. Sudden weakness, especially < moving about. Hard, ringing metallic cough, < talking, excitement, cold winds. > Eating (Anac) and drinking. Chill starts in back, shakes even near warm stove - followed by flushes of heat. < Before midnight. Hepar sulph follows well.

Sulphur	Only use in the incipient stages. Body hot, feet cold. Dullness of lungs on percussion. Increase of blood in chest. Diminished movement/respiration in upper chest, > air. Palpitations ascending. Give 1-2-3 doses high if you choose and await results. If picture comes up after tubercles have formed in the lungs be very sure of the remedy and do not repeat frequently.

Remedies particularly indicated in the later stages of TB

Arsenicum	Last stages. Do not give in the earlier stages since the disease will tend to be pushed downwards.
Baptisia	Especially useful in the later stages in relieving fever. Drowsiness, thick speech, confusion. Tongue yellow/brown centre with shiny red edges. < Afternoon.
Calc carb	Cavities form, especially right lung (Calc-p, Phos, Sep). Loud mucus rales. Soreness of chest, < touch,< pressure. Expectoration purulent, green and bloody. Hoarseness painless and persistent. Emaciation progressive. Sweats increase. Menses checked. Followed by Nit-ac.
Guiacum	Pleuritic pains, particularly left sided. Offensive sputum. A remedy in this picture that rarely fails.
Lachesis	Advanced stages, tough, green, muco-purulent expectoration. Gags, vomits mucus. Sweats especially chest, neck plus naps. Prostration (Bapt). Tongue like Bapt. Palliative.
Nit-ac	Ulceration of lungs. Hectic fever. Flushes of heat or hands and feet hot. Chilly. Loud rales. Sharp stitches. Pain extending to right scapula. Cough tickles.

Expectoration offensive, purulent, dirty green. Frequent haemorrhages of bright red blood. Dyspnoea. Hoarseness. Diarrhoea exhausts. Sweats night and early A.M. < Exertion A.M. Often indicated after Calc-c or Kali-c especially when Calc runs into debility. It prolongs life for years but does not cure.

Pix liquida 3rd stage of TB. Rales. Expectoration offensive. Pain in third left cartilage of ribs (Anisum right sided).

TB of brain:
Phos, Arg-nit, Apis, Hell.

TB of glands:
Bar-c.

TB of larynx:
Mang, (hoarseness < A.M., > Hawking). Dros, Arg-n, Arg-m.

TB of lungs:
Phos, Kali-c, Phos-ac, Lach (one of the best after pneumonia when tubercles are present). Lyc and Sil (particularly where there is liver involvement). Iodum, Oleum jecoris and Hydrastis (where there is general weakness of the stomach and diarrhoea). Spongia (characteristic dry, harsh cough often followed by Hepar which has the hard cough with much phlegm).

TB of serous membranes:
Ant-t, Ars, Bry, Hep, Phos, Kali-c.

TB of the spine
Calc-p, Caust, Bar-c.

Asthma of TB:
Dros. Mephites when Dros fails. Nat-s.

Left sided:
Mytus-c, Nat-s, Rumx, Guiacum.

All 3 lobes affected:
Sep, Calc-c, Calc-p.

Right sided:
Brom, Calc-c, Carb-an, Elaps, Kali-c, Sang.

Asthma and Rheumatism

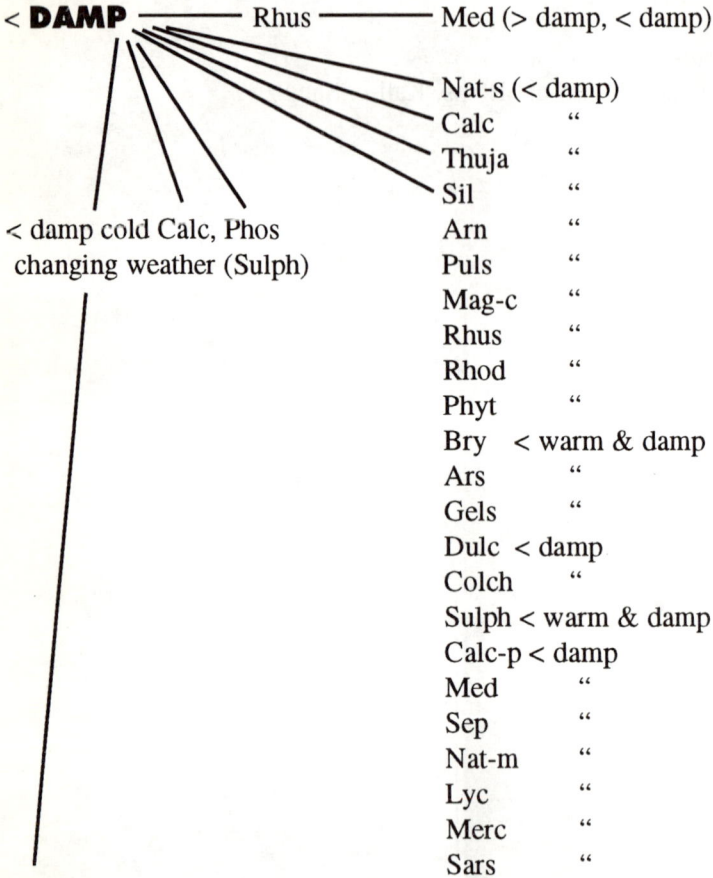

< **DAMP** ———— Rhus ———— Med (> damp, < damp)

Nat-s (< damp)
Calc   "
Thuja   "
Sil   "

< damp cold Calc, Phos   Arn   "
changing weather (Sulph)   Puls   "

Mag-c   "
Rhus   "
Rhod   "
Phyt   "
Bry   < warm & damp
Ars   "
Gels   "
Dulc   < damp
Colch   "
Sulph < warm & damp
Calc-p < damp
Med   "
Sep   "
Nat-m   "
Lyc   "
Merc   "
Sars   "

TUB - < damp, > continued motion & open air, < closed room and beginning to move. Peculiar - skin itch > heat of fire.

< *Stormy weather:*
Rhod, Phos, Sep.

Rheumatism < wet damp = pains: <*Warm:*
Bry, Calc, Carb-v, Caust, Colch,   Apis, Bry, Guaj, Iod,

Con, Dulc, Hep, Lyc, Merc, Nat-s,
Nit-ac, Phyt, Puls, Rhod, Rhus-t,
Sars, Sep, Sil, Sul, Tub, Verat,
Nux-m.

Kali-i, Ptel, Puls,
Sec, Sep, Sul, Thuj.
Merc (< warmth of bed)
Sulph   "
Phyt   "

- 28 -
Case

Two and a half years old (eight and a half years old now). Female. Blonde, sucks thumb, clear skin, reddish rosy cheeks, stocky, round stomach. Husband contradicts mother, disapproving of homœopathy.

The little girl will not speak. General slowness in most things.
She understands, nods head. Had hearing tests.
17 months considered walking. Teething at 1 year - 1st tooth.
Sitting was 5-6 months.
Very shy, quiet. Takes a long time to get used to environment.
(She was friendly with me). Very sensitive to situations.
Naturally clumsy. Cautious. Loves to read pictures.
Self contained. Introverted. Happy on her own.
Not potty trained. Loving, affectionate. Mum orientated. Loves her animal dog - this is her friend.
Bad effects after 3 inoculation jabs - fever, rash.
Birth trauma - difficult birth. Under special care.
Developed colics, evenings exactly - lasted till 10pm.
Always slept well. Nightmares, screams.
Wet patch back of head after sleep, but not now.
Feet perspire, hot feet.
No appetite, not interested, just a taste (Measles jab at 18 mths - had a good appetite till then. Feverish after jab).
Always loves her breakfast and eggs.
Throws covers off at night.
Hates changes, loves her routine.
Loves open air and being out.
A lot of colds - tendency.
Ear infection 6 months ago. Antibiotics. Nasal discharge green after this.
Terrified of doctors.

Family history:

Mother had ovarian cysts, uterine problems.
Father had surgery for testicle to be lowered.
Grandmother had a mental condition.

Repertorisation:

Slow learning to talk: Kent p.86
Agar, Bar-c, Bell, Bov, Calc, Calc-p, Caust, Nat-m, Nux-m, Sanic,
Phos, Ph-ac, Sil, Sulph.

Slow dentition: p.431
Calc, Calc-p, Phos, Sulph.

Perspiration, feet (hot):
Calc, Phos, Sulph.

Enlarged abdomen in children: p546
Calc, Sulph.

Aversion food p.481. after eating a little: Sulph.
Loves open air p.1344: Sulph.
Aversion to company, > alone: Sulph. (Tub).
Rosy cheeks, circumscribed: Sulph. (Tub).
Oversensitive, anxious p.828: Sulph.
Timidity: Sulph.
Terrified of doctors: (Tub)

Sulphur 30. To be repeated again if appetite not improved. Needed
to repeat in a week, Sulphur 30.

Had an acute cold with pain in the ears - lasted 2 and a half hours.
After cold finished, Sulphur 200.

Now three years old - had a small bite from a dog. Went into a hysterical shock. Wanting to be carried. Diarrhoea. Started to wet bed
(dry previously). Aconite 30.

Then refused to bathe. Shivered from fright. Repeated Sulphur 200.

Starting to talk, actually putting words together.
Cries if mother laughs (Tub). (Offended easily, frightened).
Fear of people. Very clumsy. Still a very quiet child.
A lot more general life in her.
Now starts climbing in the play group.
Feet more sweaty and odorous.

Sulphur 200.

Appetite much improved but limited.
She's happier being with the father now!
Still cautious, not adventurous. Odorous vaginal discharge.
Stubborness developing strongly - angers. Can only persuade her to do something if it's her idea. Then she will do it.
Only kisses with her forehead as a touch. If anyone tries to hug her she pulls away. Dislikes contact or touch, it irritates. Beginning to hit out if frustrated. This is becoming much more obvious. Now wants to remain outside only and play at silent games with her silent dog.

Sulphur 1M.

Not the expected change. Angers and hitting out more apparent.

Tuberculinum 200.

Feet sweaty, odorous.
Food - tends to be fussy, but tries new things. Loves cheese all day.
Loves sourness, chocolate cake. Slow eater - takes ages. Loves ice cream (Tub).
Now will only kiss her mother - no one else!
More adventurous. Talking much more.
Still concerned if people laugh.

Tuberculinum 200.

4 years of age. At school all day. Quiet. Feels more energetic. Speech needs correction. Plays well in a group. Relates to only one person. A loner.
Much less frightened. Still fearful of noise.
Leucorrhoea.
Eats more quickly.
Timid, quiet, introverted.
Tuberculinum 1M.

Needs reassurance, lacks confidence.
Will kiss anyone now. Feet warm and sweaty.
Less fearful. Still very sensitive about a lot of things.
Epistaxis - new symptom.
Threadworms periodically.
Upset easily if repremanded. Thrives on complements.
Speech fine. Reading fine.

Five years of age.

Improvement did not last as well as before.
Lacks stamina. No colds. No vaginal thrush.
Very sensitive to atmospheres and people - gets very excitable and agitated.
Reprimands are a personal attack resulting in major tantrums.

(Mother) Did not say that earlier on she got feverish, 104°. Cold and tickling cough. Tonsilitis. In desperation parents refered to GP. Amoxyl - 5 day course.
She got over this feverish bout quickly.
But she seems to have become more obsessive.
Improved in energy.

Tuberculinum 1M. Lasted 4 months.

Six years of age.

Had an attack of 'flu.
Can't use her legs - crawls as if muscles siezed up. Legs ache, very stiff in the mornings, < after moving about.
Still a loner.
Shakey. Tremors. Stomachache.
Temperature 101°. Can't shake off this fever.
Talking regressed.

Talking confused nonsense Kent p.81-82: Tub.
Stiffness after exertion p.1191: Arn, Calc-c, Rhus-t, Tub.

Tuberculinum 10M.

Did very well. No contact for over a year.
She has had yet another cold. Started suddenly with fever. Hot. Sore throat.

Belladonna 200.

Chronic treatment was resumed after this acute attack and an amelioration continued on the Tuberculinum.

Conclusion

To quote from Kent's Materia Medica p949:

"I do not use Tuberculinum merely because it is a nosode, or with the idea that generally prevails of using nosodes; that is a product of the disease for the disease, and the results of the disease... It is hoped... that we may be able to prescribe Tuberculinum on the symptoms of Tuberculinum just as we would use any other drug. It is deep acting, constitutionally deep... it is long acting, and it affects the constitutions more deeply than most remedies; and when our deepest remedies act only a few weeks, and they have to be changed, this remedy comes in as one of the remedies - when symptoms agree - and brings a better state of reaction, so that remedies hold longer."

Tuberculinum is a much needed remedy which is a combination of the psoric and syphilitic miasms. Sometimes the psoric side is stronger, at other times the syphilitic side is uppermost and active. First the dissatisfied, restless, fatigue of the psoric, then the emaciation and tubercular destructive deposits on the lungs or the crippling knee joints of the syphilitic side.

We are indeed indebted to the provers for this remedy, for in practice it is so often indicated.

- 30 -
Glossary

Antidote:
The next most similar remedy chosen to match the presenting symptoms. This modifies the effect of the first given if there is an excessive over reaction.

Intercurrent remedies:
There are phases of acute conditions which call for a remedy, eg. injuries, flu' or emergencies, which may differ from the constitutional remedy given.

Miasm:
Is a German word that is not possible to translate. Today the best word we may use is a pre-disposition in the constitution of the person. Miasms are inherited, the psoric, syphilitic and sycotic.

Nosode:
Is a remedy made from a disease product. After provings we are able to use them as any other remedy according to the similar.

Pseudo-psora:
In some books it is actually the tubercular miasm.

Psora:
The original interior disturbance of mankind. From a perfect state of existence within his environment man became anxious (for example). These various changes progressed and the first states of susceptibility to the environment became manifest. These inner changes showed in mans adaptability.

Sycosis:
In chronological order the gonococcus of the venereal disease appeared later. This became the 'pattern' of the inherited disease. But sycosis is more complicated for vaccinations, immunisations and suppressed discharges as non-specific urethritis all manifest chronically in a sycotic 'pattern'. We therefore have two forms.

Syphilis:
The original venereal disease manifesting as far as is known after psora. It was the scourge of Europe from the 11th century onwards and it spread. It has its characteristic signs and symptoms, its secondary and tertiary stages. This is the acquired disease. After medical treatment acquired syphilis becomes a chronic state. The 'pattern' manifests as symptoms. This is miasmatic as the pattern can be inherited by many generations.

Tubercular:
Is an inherited miasm which has a 'pattern' of the psoric - syphilitic combination.

Relationship of remedies:
Certain remedies follow each other well especially if the case shows that other remedies will be needed later.One remedy completes a cure which the other begins. The relationship of remedies, or cognates as Kent states, need to be known

bd: Twice daily.

tds: Three times daily.